Decision–Making in Operative Dentistry

Quintessentials of Dental Practice – 3
Operative Dentistry - 1

Decision–Making in Operative Dentistry

By
Paul A Brunton

Editor-in-Chief: Nairn H F Wilson
Editor Operative Dentistry: Paul A Brunton

Quintessence Publishing Co. Ltd.

London, Berlin, Chicago, Copenhagen, Paris, Milan, Barcelona,
Istanbul, São Paulo, Tokyo, New Dehli, Moscow, Prague, Warsaw

British Library Cataloguing in Publication Data

Brunton, Paul A.
  Decision-making in operative dentistry. – (The quintessentials of dental practice)
  1. Dentistry, Operative – Decision making
  I. Title II. Wilson, Nairn H. F.
  617.6′05

  ISBN 1850970572

ISBN 1-85097-057-2

Foreword

It is widely accepted that more that 60 per cent of a general dental practitioner's time is spent practising operative dentistry, predominantly the replacement of restorations. Central to success in this major element of everyday practice is effective decision-making. Realising that goal is difficult given limitations in many of the existing diagnostic systems and techniques – and the lack of consensus in respect of criteria for certain forms of operative intervention. Moreover, the existing literature gives mixed messages – for example, in relation to the use of liners, bases and sealers.

In addressing questions frequently posed by practitioners, *Decision-Making in Operative Dentistry* – Volume 3 of the Quintessentials for General Practitioners Series – is highly relevant to the modern practice of dentistry. For practitioners not yet introduced to the concepts of minimal intervention, the repair and refurbishment of restorations, and conservative techniques for the management of tooth wear, this book will be a revelation. For colleagues familiar with such concepts, *Decision-Making in Operative Dentistry* will be an invaluable guide to the "when, where and how" of the modern patient-centred approach to the conservation of teeth. Written in the succinct, easy-to-read style that characterises the Quintessentials for General Dental Practitioners Series, this book will not fail to give the busy practitioner new knowledge and insight that can be immediately applied to the benefit of patients. For practitioners who think that operative dentistry has not really changed since they were a student, this book is indispensable reading.

Nairn Wilson
Editor-in-Chief

Preface

This book does not seek to provide the reader with comprehensive coverage of the subject of operative dentistry. There are already several excellent textbooks available that have addressed the subject in depth, particularly from the undergraduate's perspective.

This book is about the practice of contemporary operative dentistry in primary dental care. Its principal aim is to assist clinical decision-making in the dental surgery and provide answers to the questions practitioners frequently ask. As such, the approach to the subject is very different and somewhat novel.

Preservative operative dentistry is the philosophy on which this book is based. The continued use of amalgam, particularly for initial lesion management, does not sit well with this philosophy. Amalgam has, however, been included in this edition to ensure comprehensive coverage. I suspect that future editions will not cover or support the continued use of amalgam.

The classification of lesions of caries has changed in recent years. Accordingly, I have not used Black's classification, preferring to classify lesions as occlusal, proximal and cervical. Similarly, the FDI system of tooth notation has been used. On a final note, this book considers the restoration of the adult dentition with direct restorative materials and techniques. Readers will be aware that operative dentistry includes the provision of single-unit indirect restorations, which is outside the remit of this publication.

On reading this book the reader will be able to:
- diagnose caries more effectively, especially in its early stages
- intervene appropriately and only when absolutely necessary
- prepare teeth minimally and effectively
- select the correct restorative material
- understand modern pulp protection regimes
- select restorations suitable for repair and refurbishment procedures
- identify and treat non-carious tooth tissue loss.

Paul A Brunton

Acknowledgements

The author would like to thank Drs Andrew Bristow, Paul McCabe, Leean Morrow, David Simpkins, Chris Sweet, Ian Wood and Professor David Watts for reviewing the entire manuscript and providing valuable feedback.

The author is also indebted to the following individuals and publishers who have generously provided illustrations which have made the publication of this book possible. Figs 1-6–1-9: Dr Denise Cortes, Gama Filho University, Brazil; Figs 1-5 and 1-16: Dr Roger Ellwood; Figs 1-11 and 1-12: Dr Viv Rushton; Fig 1-15: KaVo (UK) Ltd.; Fig 4-5: Professor Nairn Wilson; Figs 4-6–4-13: reproduced with kind permission of Independent Dentistry; Figs 6-2–6-6, 6-9–6-12, 6-13–6-18: reproduced with kind permission of Quintessenz Verlag, Berlin; Figs 7-2–7-4: Ms Leean Morrow; and Figs 7-6, 7-8 and 7-9: reproduced with kind permission of FDI World Press Ltd.

Contents

Chapter 1

Clinical Diagnosis of Dental Caries. Is it Caries?

Aim

With changing patterns of disease experience the diagnosis of caries, particularly in its early stages, continues to be difficult for clinicians. The aim of this chapter is to improve understanding of modern methods of caries diagnosis.

Outcome

Practitioners will be familiar with modern methods of detecting dental caries and their relevance to contemporary dental practice.

Introduction

The pattern of dental caries has changed in recent years, with smooth surface lesions becoming less common and new lesions more likely to develop in pits and fissures. It is arguably easier to diagnose early caries on smooth surfaces (with the exception of proximal surfaces) than in pits and fissures, particularly when occult occlusal caries is present. In this condition the tooth can appear sound when examined visually but on radiographic examination there is extensive caries affecting the dentine (Fig 1-1).

Diagnostic Tests

With all diagnostic tests there is potential for operator error. For example, four outcomes are possible when a diagnostic test is applied to detect caries. These are as follows:

True positive
This occurs when caries is present and the test correctly identifies this. A good diagnostic test will have a high percentage of true positive outcomes.

False positive
A false positive result occurs when a diagnostic test incorrectly identifies caries when caries is not present.

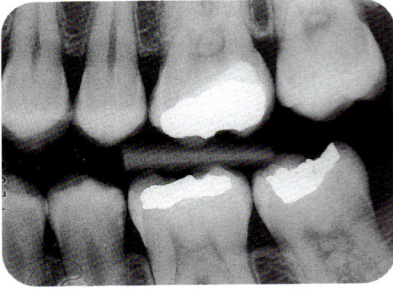

Fig 1-1 Radiograph showing caries as follows: mesial 16, distal and mesial 15, distal 45, mesial and distal 46 and mesial 47.

True negative
This outcome is the opposite of a true positive result. It occurs when the test correctly identifies an individual as caries free and they are, in fact, free of the condition.

False negative
If a patient has caries and the test incorrectly deems them to be caries free then the outcome is defined as false negative.

These four possible outcomes of a diagnostic test are summarised in Fig 1-2.

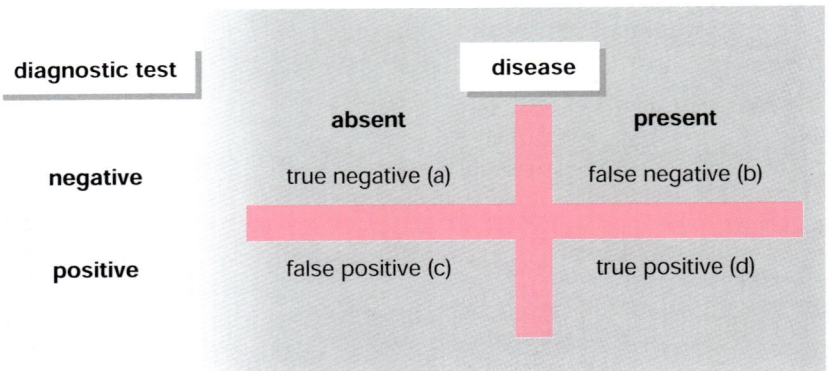

Fig 1-2 Diagrammatic representation of diagnostic test outcomes.

Table 1-1 The sensitivity and specificity of diagnostic tests commonly used to detect dental caries.

Test	Sensitivity	Specificity
Visual examination	0.38	0.99
Transillumination	0.67	0.97
Radiographs	0.59	0.96
Laser	0.76–0.87	0.72–0.87
Electrical conductance	0.80–0.97	0.56–0.89

Sensitivity and Specificity

Sensitivity and specificity are both measures of how accurate a diagnostic test is in terms of its ability correctly to identify individuals as diseased and non-diseased. *Sensitivity* is defined as the proportion of true positives that are correctly identified. It is calculated as follows (true negative = a, false negative = b, false positive = c, true positive = d):

$$\text{sensitivity} = \frac{100d}{(b + d)}$$

The numbers of true positives and false negatives are related numerically; hence the proportion of true positive results for a diagnostic test (sensitivity) is 1 minus the false negative rate.

Specificity is the proportion of correctly identified true negative results and this is 1 minus the false positive rate. It is calculated as follows:

$$\text{specificity} = \frac{100a}{(a + c)}$$

A good diagnostic test would have both high specificity and high sensitivity, which means the number of times the test is likely to give an incorrect result is low. In practice, as the level of either sensitivity or specificity rises, the other falls, so a balance must be struck.

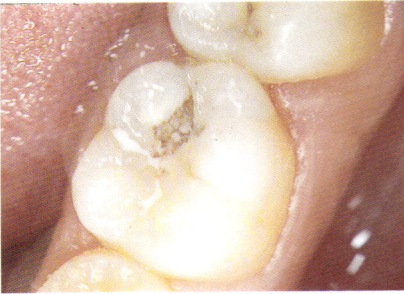

Fig 1-3 Frank occlusal caries with cavitation in 36.

The sensitivity and specificity of diagnostic tests commonly used to detect dental caries are shown in Table 1-1.

Visual Examination

Visual examination of a tooth is the most widely used method of diagnosing dental caries. This method is, however, incredibly inaccurate. The use of a probe, blunt or otherwise, is contraindicated as it is a poor test of the presence of caries and likely to cause cavitation of an early demineralised lesion. Probes should therefore be used to remove soft depo-sits only during a clinical examination.

Whilst cavitation is quite easy to diagnose, looking for discolouration, which is suggestive of caries, is more difficult (Fig 1-3). The operator's ability to see discolouration depends on the nature and direction of the illumination and whether magnification is used or not. Radiographs are useful aids in con-

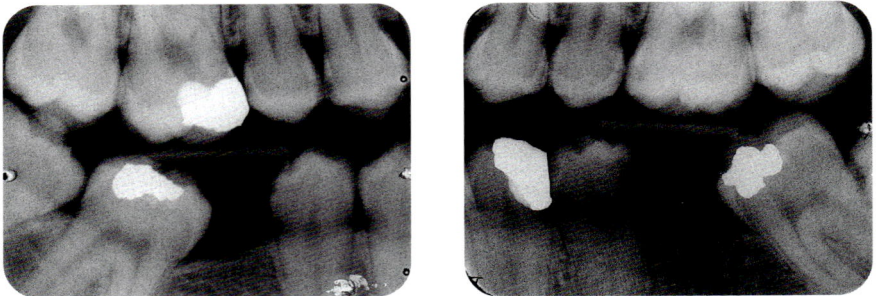

Fig 1-4 Radiographs of a new patient, which emphasize the benefit of baseline bitewing radiography.

firming a clinical suspicion of caries, especially proximal caries (Fig 1-4). When radiographs are used to confirm the presence of occlusal caries, however, superimposition of the cuspal pattern can be a problem, which makes their use for detecting early occlusal caries somewhat limited.

Transillumination

This technique uses an intense beam of white light to transilluminate the tooth (Fig 1-5). The tip of the light is placed on the buccal or lingual surface of the tooth and as caries has a lower index of transmitted light it shows as darkening of the tooth (Figs 1-6–1-7). This technique can be used to detect proximal caries in anterior teeth and selected posterior teeth and may be useful in the diagnosis of cracked tooth syndrome (Figs 1-8 –1-9).

The light units used for transillumination typically have an output of 2,000 lux generated from a 150 watt lamp with a tip diameter of 0.5 mm. The units are relatively inexpensive and, given the increasing number of fibre optic handpieces, it would be feasible to have a fibre optic tip attached to dental

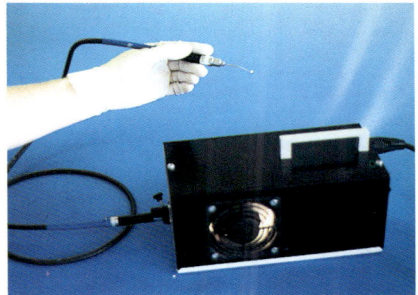

Fig 1-5 Light for transillumination of teeth.

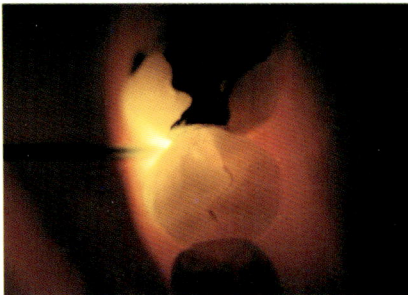

Fig 1-6 Transillumination of distal aspect of 35 showing distal caries.

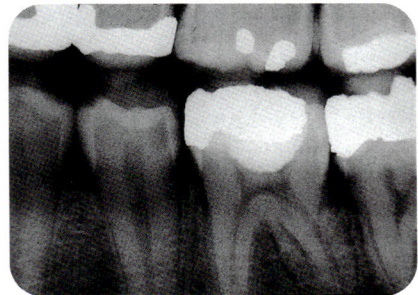

Fig 1-7 Radiograph confirming presence of caries distally in 35.

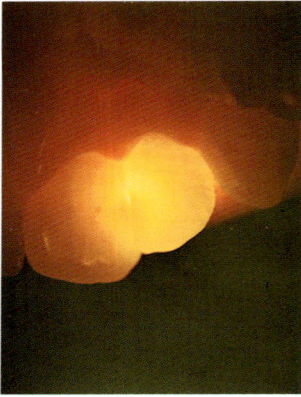

Fig 1-8 Transillumination of 21 and 22 showing caries distally in 21 and mesially in 22.

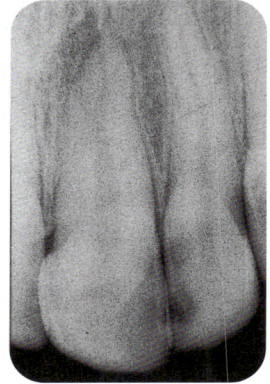

Fig 1-9 Radiograph confirming presence of caries distally in 21 and mesially in 22 detected by transillumination.

units. Special equipment is not required for the transillumination of anterior teeth. The beam of light from the operating light can be redirected with a hand mirror to transilluminate anterior teeth. The high sensitivity seen with this technique, arguably greater than when radiographs are used, offers practitioners a promising non-interventive technique for caries diagnosis.

Radiography

Radiographs are useful for the following:
• To confirm a clinical suspicion of proximal caries.
• To detect early non-cavitated proximal lesions, which are amenable to preventive care.
• For serial monitoring of lesions to look for evidence of disease activity.
• To provide an indication of the size and extent of the lesion, remembering that clinically the lesion will always be more extensive.

The aim when using radiographs is really to separate lesions, if present, into those which require restorative therapy as distinct from those which will respond to preventive regimes (Fig 1-10).

For the detection of caries, intraoral radiographs, specifically bitewing radiographs for posterior teeth and periapical radiographs for anterior teeth, are

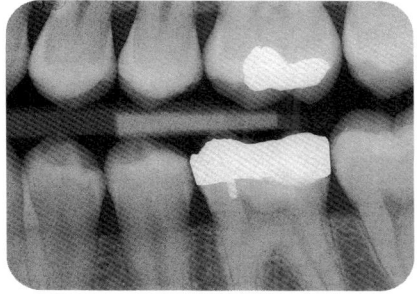

Fig 1-10 Radiograph showing lesions to be monitored in distal of 24 and mesial 25 and one which requires restorative therapy in distal of 35.

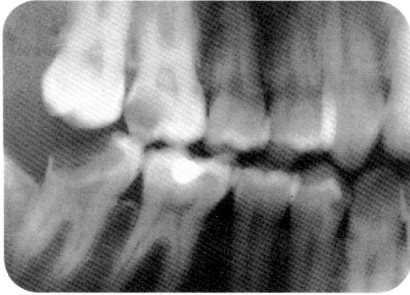

Fig 1-11 Part of a DPT suggesting caries is present in mesial of 44.

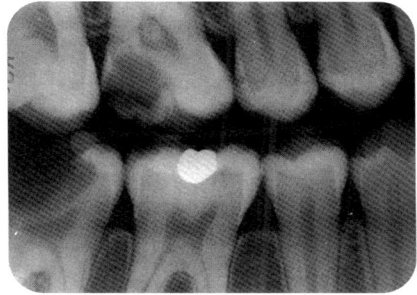

Fig 1-12 Intra-oral radiograph, which confirms that 44 is sound.

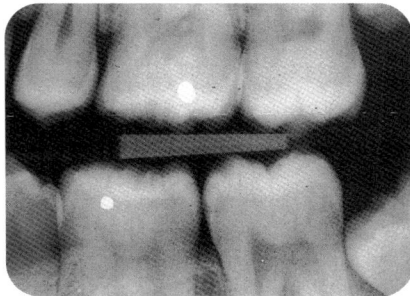

Fig 1-13 Bitewing radiograph of 37 showing a mesial lesion in a low-caries-risk individual.

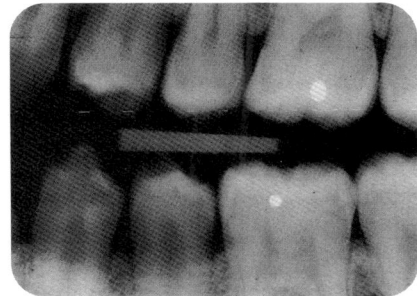

Fig 1-14 Bitewing of 37 taken six months later showing the lesion has not progressed and is currently not active.

the only radiographs that should be used. Extraoral radiographs (for example, panoramic radiographs) have no place in the diagnosis of caries, as they can be misleading and wildly inaccurate (Figs 1-11–1-12).

All new patients should have bitewing radiographs taken at their first appointment to confirm the presence or absence of dental caries and to give an indication of bone levels. These radiographs act as a baseline against which other radiographs can be compared. The interval before repeat radiographs are taken depends primarily on the caries risk assessment of the patient. This gives the practitioner a guide as to whether lesions are progressing (Figs 1-13–1-14). To facilitate comparisons with subsequent radiographs, all bitewing radiographs should be taken with a film holder, which will make the beam angulation used more consistent. The use of faster films, which result in less radiation exposure to the patient, has resulted in radiographs which are not as sharp as slower films. This makes identification of early lesions more demanding, although the use of an x-ray magnifier is helpful. It is, however, difficult ethically to justify the use of slower films when faster films are available and it is recommended that practitioners consider changing to faster films for this reason.

The advent of digital radiography in conjunction with diagnostic software is a potentially useful development. This method does not use a film but a storage phosphor plate, which is the size of a conventional film. The plate is exposed as for a conventional film and placed into a reader, which is attached to a computer. Another system uses a charge coupler device connected directly to a computer. The advantage of these systems is that they are low dose and the image is almost instantaneous. The cost of such systems, however, is high. The system can be matched with caries-detection software, based on subtraction radiography, which detects early lesions and could potentially compare serial images to give information on lesion progression. These systems are in the early stages of their development and further evaluation is needed.

Lasers

Lasers have recently been introduced to assist practitioners in caries diagnosis, especially in diagnosing early enamel lesions (Fig 1-15). The concept is based on laser fluorescence in that caries illuminated by a laser will fluoresce and the degree to which this occurs is an indication of the extent of the disease process. The laser is directed into the fissure and the two-way handpiece allows the unit to quantify the reflected laser light energy simultane-

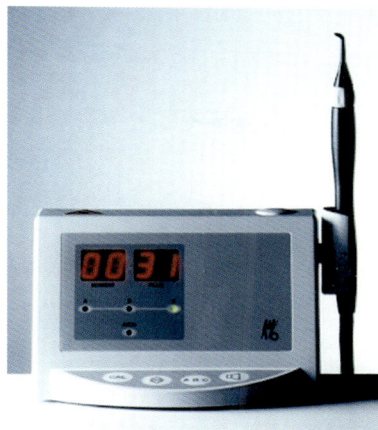

Fig 1-15 Laser-based diagnostic system.

ously. The wavelength of the light used is such that normal unaffected enamel exhibits little or no fluorescence. The feedback from the handpiece is translated to an analogue scale, with a low reading indicating a sound tooth. Increasingly higher readings indicate preventive therapy, monitoring, placement of a fissure sealant or restoration respectively. Heavily stained fissures are problematic and the system, it would appear, is only useful for occlusal lesions.

Electrical Conduction Methods

Diagnostic techniques based on electrical conductance have been used in dentistry since the late 1950s. The techniques were based on the premise that sound enamel is a good electrical insulator. Teeth affected by caries develop porosities, which fill with water and ions from saliva. As the lesion develops these porosities coalesce forming pathways that allow the passage of an electric current, resulting in a drop in electrical resistance. The degree by which the resistance drops is a good indicator of caries development. Commercial systems have been developed and marketed based on this principle. The technique was never widely adopted by practitioners owing to its inherent limitations, which included the need to dry the tooth and then wet the fissures with saline to facilitate conductance. Further research has shown that the use of electrical resistance measurements in caries diagnosis is more accurate than visual examination and this has led to a renewed interest in this technique.

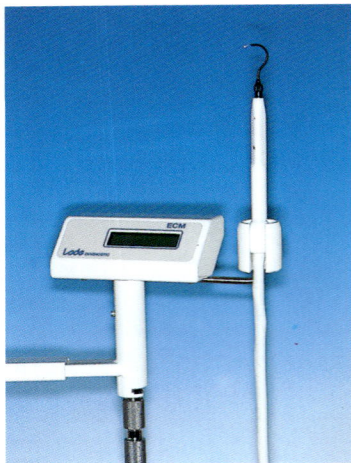

Fig 1-16 Electronic caries meter.

An electronic caries meter is now available which has an air flow system that dries the tooth (Fig 1-16). The meter has been shown to be very accurate in detecting early lesions. A disadvantage of the technique is that it can incorrectly identify a significant number (over 40%) of surfaces as diseased when they are sound, i.e. a low specificity. This is not a problem provided the technique is used to identify early lesions and to monitor lesion progression rather than indicate intervention is required. Lesions which are just into dentine are typically not cavitated and therefore do not warrant intervention. The system is very helpful in identifying lesions that would benefit from preventive measures, whilst visual examination and radiographs are better predictors of whether operative intervention is indicated.

Recommended Reading

Faculty of General Dental Practitioners. Selection Criteria for Dental Radiography. London: Royal College of Surgeons of England, 1998.

Chapter 2
Caries Risk Assessment and Criteria for Intervention. When Should You Intervene?

Aim

Deciding when to restore a carious cavity and when to monitor a lesion has historically been largely subjective and prone to substantial variation between practitioners. The aim of this chapter is to provide objective criteria that a practitioner can use to decide as to when operative intervention is indicated.

Outcome

After completing this section practitioners will be familiar with caries risk assessment and how the caries risk assessment of a patient weights the decision to intervene or not, as the case may be. Similarly, objective criteria are discussed which can be applied to individual lesions to assist practitioners in deciding to intervene more appropriately.

Introduction

A decision when to intervene in the management of caries is probably amongst the most important decisions a dentist makes. Tooth preparation is irreversible and places the tooth on the restorative staircase. Eventually all restorations fail and where repair and refurbishment procedures cannot usefully extend the life of the restoration, a replacement (typically, larger) restoration will be required. Inevitably when failed restorations are removed and replaced, more tooth tissue is lost and the preparation becomes more extensive, possibly requiring a cuspal coverage indirect restoration, which requires further tooth reduction. At some point on the restorative staircase it is likely that the pulp becomes involved. It is crucial, therefore, that operative intervention should be delayed until indicated clinically or absolutely necessary and the nature of the intervention should be limited to preserve tooth tissue but also to prolong the life of the restored unit.

When Should You Intervene?

Until relatively recently, the threshold for operative intervention was held to be: when a carious cavity was shown to be in dentine radiographically or when the lesion was visibly cavitated. If these criteria were adopted universally, arrested or static lesions would be restored unnecessarily. Consequently, it is now the accepted convention that lesions are restored if they are into dentine and there is evidence that they are progressing. Cavitated lesions continue, by definition, to require restoration. Operative management of lesions extending into dentine is favoured in patients who have a high or medium risk of developing new lesions.

Caries Risk Status

Caries risk assessment is defined as the risk that a patient will develop new lesions of caries or existing lesions will continue to progress, assuming that all aetiological factors (diet, time, susceptible surface and plaque levels) remain equal. It is an important assessment as it helps a clinician to decide whether to monitor or to restore caries. It also influences the recall period for patients in regular dental care, let alone the frequency that further radiographs should be taken for monitoring purposes. Patients are assessed as being at high, medium and low risk of developing further lesions. It is important to accept that patients can change their caries-risk status – moving from low to high by changing their diet (for example, students leaving home and altering their diet, older patients, patients post radiotherapy, or past smokers sucking sweets more frequently than normal to combat the effects of a dry mouth or in place of a cigarette).

Determining Risk

The following factors influence the caries risk for an individual patient:
- The patient's diet, especially if the diet is rich in fermentable carbohydrates, i.e. cariogenic.
- The frequency of consumption of fermentable carbohydrates.
- The presence and amount of cariogenic bacteria, specifically lactobacillus and streptococcus mutans, in the plaque biofilm.
- Saliva—both the amount (volume) and buffering capacity (quality).
- Socio-economic status and social history. Caries is a disease of deprivation and therefore patients with low socio-economic status are more likely to develop new lesions and existing lesions are more likely to progress.

Table 2-1 Determination of caries risk.

Factor		High	Low
Diet	diet history	diet high in fermentablele carbohydrates	diet low in fermentablele carbohydrates
Frequency	frequency of consumption with diet history	frequent consumption not confined to mealtimes	infrequent consumption or confined to mealtimes
Plaque	amount and nature	high plaque score	low plaque score
Saliva	amount and nature	low flow rates high lactobacilli and streptococcus counts	high flow rates low lactobacilli and streptococcus counts
Socio-economic status		not dentally motivated;	dentally motivated patients;
		deprived background; low dental aspirations; high caries family	privileged background; high dental aspirations; low caries family
Past disease experience		high number of filled and missing surfaces (FMS)	low number of filled and missing surfaces (FMS)
Current disease experience		high number of decayed surfaces (DS)	low number of decayed surfaces (DS)
Attendance pattern		irregular and or pain-only attenders	regular attenders
Fluoride and Chlorhexidine		infrequent use of rinses and toothpaste; non-fluoridated water supply	frequent use of rinses and toothpastes; fluoridated water supply
Medical history		xerostomia; learning difficulties; cariogenic medication	fit and well
Other		partial dentures used to replace missing units	bridgework used to replace missing units

- Previous disease experience—which is usually assessed by the number of restorations, although it may mean that the patient has previously attended a practitioner with a low intervention threshold. Other useful indicators are missing teeth, i.e. not those removed for orthodontic reasons.
- Current disease experience (for example, the number of "white spot" lesions and the presence of cavitated lesions).
- Attendance pattern. Regular attenders are likely to have a lower risk assigned than more infrequent attenders, where monitoring of teeth is not feasible.
- Fluoride and chlorhexidine use.
- Systemic illness of dental significance.

Several computer programs have been written to assist the practitioner in assessing the caries risk of patients. These initiatives may be considered to be in their infancy and to need further evaluation before they can be recommended for routine use. It is easy, however, to foresee a time when caries risk assessment programs will be used routinely alongside digital radiography to assist practitioners in managing dental caries more effectively.

Until these systems are widely available and validated, it is suggested that the above factors are considered to determine the caries risk for a patient. A high-risk category would be allocated to a patient where the majority of the factors above point to a high risk and vice versa. Moderate risk would be attributed where the factors in Table 2-1 balance out. It is crucial to explain to the patient the importance of these factors. Your shared agenda should be to work to reduce the factors to those of low risk wherever possible. Table 2-2 shows how caries risk assessment affects recall frequency, intervention and radiographic monitoring.

In the following section, occlusal, proximal and cervical caries will be considered separately. Objective guidance is given to assist practitioners in assessing individual lesions to determine if operative intervention is indicated or whether monitoring is more appropriate. In individuals with a moderate caries risk it may be appropriate to monitor certain lesions whilst restoring others.

Occlusal Caries

The occlusal surface of the dried tooth should be carefully examined after a prophylaxis and the decision made as to whether the occlusal surface is:

Table 2-2 Caries risk assessment.

Caries risk	Recall interval	Intervention	Radiograph frequency
High	6-monthly	yes	6-monthly
Moderate	6- to 12-monthly	yes	12-monthly
Low	12- to 24-monthly	monitor	12- to 24-monthly

- sound
- stained
- stained and decalcified
- visibly cavitated.

During this examination, probes should not be used except to remove debris. As noted above, probing fissures that are in the early stages of demineralisation will result in disruption to the enamel matrix and cause cavitation at the expense of remineralisation.

The management options for occlusal caries include the following (see Fig 2-1):
- monitoring and instituting preventive regimes
- fissure sealant
- preventive resin restoration
- resin composite or amalgam restoration.

Sound fissure
No treatment is required if the patient has a low caries risk and/or the tooth has been erupted for more than two years. If the tooth is within two years of eruption and the patient has a high or medium caries risk, and/or their dental management is complicated by a medical condition (for example, haemophilia or moderate to severe learning difficulties, where future management would be complicated), a fissure sealant is indicated.

Stained fissure
No active treatment is required if the patient has no active caries and there is no radiographic evidence of dentinal caries. If the patient has a high to medium risk of developing further lesions then fissure sealants are indicated, especially if the teeth are within two years of eruption.

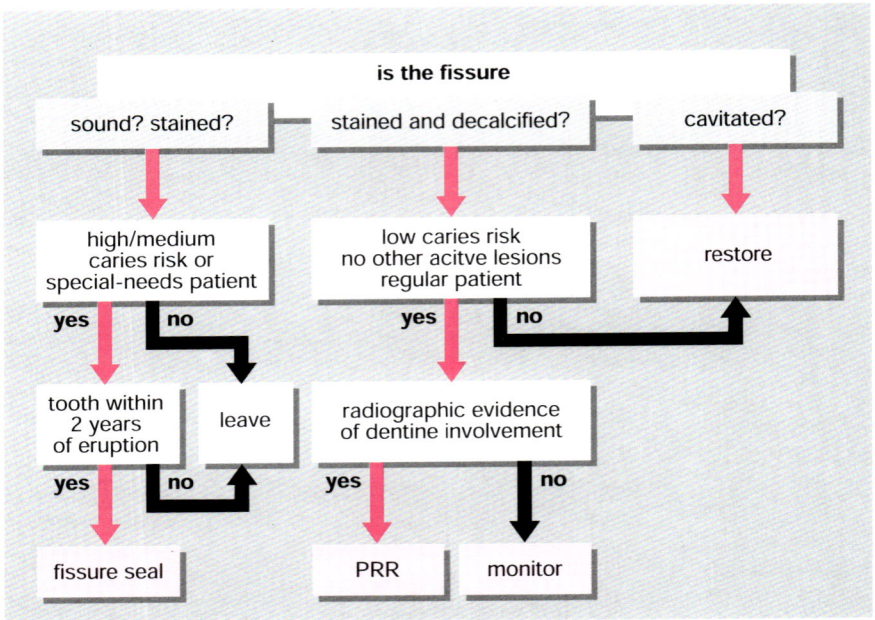

Fig 2-1 Algorithm for the management of occlusal caries.

Stained and decalcified fissure
Fissures that are stained and decalcified should be monitored in the following circumstances:
• No other active lesions are diagnosed and the patient's risk of developing new lesions is assessed to be low.
• There is no radiographic evidence of dentinal caries. If there is limited radiographic evidence of dentinal caries then a preventive resin restoration is indicated.
• Reliable patient on regular review.

Cavitation
Always requires restoration. However, a small cavity in a complex fissure pattern that extends into dentine after caries removal is best treated with a preventive resin restoration.

Proximal caries
Diagnosis is generally complicated by the lack of visual access to assess the surface of the tooth for cavitation. The practitioner is therefore reliant on

radiographs for the diagnosis and assessment of proximal lesions. Given that proximal lesions progress slowly, it is now accepted that lesions of proximal caries have to have progressed at least through the outer third of dentine before a proximal lesion will have cavitated. Intervention is therefore indicated, in a low-risk patient, when a proximal lesion has passed the amelo-dentinal junction (ADJ) and has been shown to be progressing by serial radiographs. It is only acceptable to monitor lesions in this way provided the number of lesions monitored is weighed against the caries risk of the patient who is in regular ongoing dental care. Intervention is indicated, however, when a lesion has reached the ADJ in moderate- and high-risk patients (see Fig 2-2).

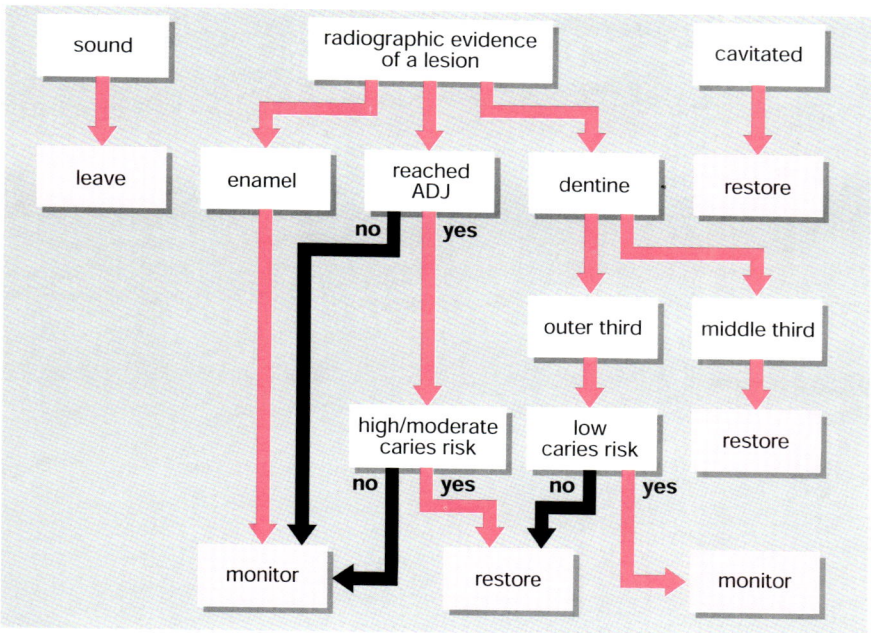

Fig 2-2 Algorithm for the management of proximal caries.

Cervical caries

Cervical surfaces can be sound, stained, stained and decalcified or cavitated, and again the operator must be able to distinguish between the latter three conditions without the use of a probe except to remove debris. Generally, surfaces which are stained should be monitored, whilst surfaces which are stained and decalcified should be encouraged to remineralise and the lesion arrested by recommending the adjunctive use of fluoride and chlorhexidine mouthwashes. Cavitated lesions require operative intervention (Fig 2-3).

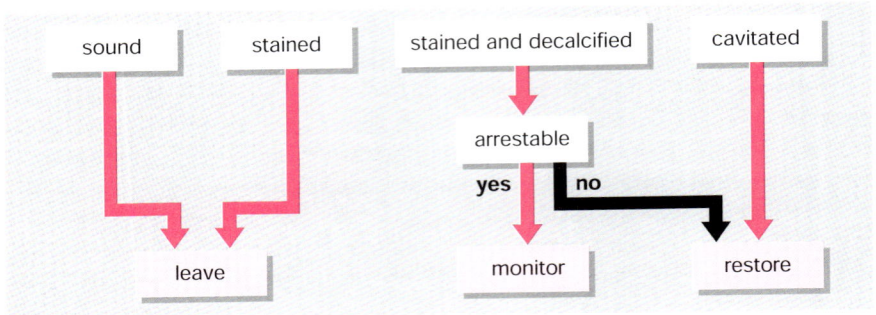

Fig 2-3 Algorithm for the management of cervical caries.

Recommended Reading

Anusavice KJ. Management of dental caries as a chronic infectious disease. J Dent-Educ 1998;62:791–802.

Chapter 3

Preservative Operative Intervention. How to Intervene?

Aim

Deciding how best to intervene and prepare teeth if operative management of dental caries is indicated is an everyday scenario for the practitioner. The aim of this chapter is to consider several techniques for preparing teeth for the placement of a direct restoration.

Outcome

This section familiarises practitioners with:
- how to intervene and prepare teeth
- traditional tooth preparation techniques
- micro-preparation techniques
- chemomechanical methods of caries removal
- sonic tooth preparation
- air abrasion
- the use of magnification.

Tooth Preparation

The general overriding principle when operative intervention is indicated is that ideally the preparation should be only as large as the lesion itself. It is anticipated that the strict requirement to remove all caries (i.e. affected but uninfected dentine) is changing, although it is currently accepted practice to remove all softened dentine and to ensure the amelodentinal junction (ADJ) is clear of caries once tooth preparation is complete.

Occlusal preparation
Information about the extent and depth of the lesion can be gained from any pre-operative radiographs that are available. Whilst this is useful, it is important to remember that this is always an under-representation of the true extent of the lesion. The lesion is accessed with a bur and the preparation extended until all affected fissures have been removed and the ADJ appears normal,

with no visual evidence of caries. Sound fissures are not removed and if two lesions are present they are treated separately.

Fissures that are decalcified but not cavitated at the edge of the lesion can be left and fissure sealed after the restoration has been placed, or as part of the restorative process. If amalgam is used, a cavosurface margin of 90–110° is required. Undermined enamel at the margins should be removed, as the restorative material will not support it, with possible fracture subsequently. In contrast, preparations for resin composite require the removal of friable enamel only, as unsupported, but firm enamel can be supported by the restorative material and may be left.

Bevels at the margins of the preparation are contraindicated for either material as they result in thin sections of the material at the preparation margin. These can fracture off under normal occlusal loading, providing a niche for stain build-up or acting as a plaque-retention factor. Another practitioner might misdiagnose these stained marginal fractures as secondary caries and replace the restoration unnecessarily.

Fissure sealing of minimal occlusal resin composite restorations is good practice and places the unaffected fissures out of reach of further carious attack if the sealant is placed carefully. Any early initial caries in the fissure will "burn out" as further substrate in the form of fermentable carbohydrate is denied to the lesion. It has also been shown that there is some advantage in terms of enhanced longevity to fissure-sealing teeth after amalgam restorations have been placed using an unfilled resin system.

In theory, amalgam restorations require an undercut to retain them and traditionally this was built into preparations with inverted cone burs. In practice, if fissure burs are used, the nylon chuck of the modern air turbine handpiece allows the bur to rotate eccentrically and undercut is automatically incorporated into the preparation during tooth preparation. It is preferable, however, to use a small pear-shaped bur, which will by its very nature preserve occlusal tissue and build in undercuts. A pear-shaped bur has a shape similar to that of the lesion of caries. The continued use of inverted cone burs will further weaken cusps in teeth with large occlusal and/or proximal preparations, especially if there are buccal and lingual or palatal extensions to the preparation. Consequently, their continued use cannot be justified.

Proximal preparations in posterior teeth
Lesions of proximal caries in posterior teeth are notoriously difficult to treat,

especially at the initial stage, with damage to adjacent teeth relatively common when proximal lesions are prepared with traditional techniques. It is important to distinguish between occlusal and proximal preparations in that a proximal preparation may have an occlusal dimension, but frequently there is no occlusal caries. The belief that occlusal dovetails are required for retention of proximal amalgam restorations is no longer valid. Whilst adjacent occlusal and proximal lesions that have coalesced in premolar teeth are often treated together for convenience, this is not the case for permanent molar teeth in that a lower molar may have up to four restorations: namely, one or two proximal and one or two occlusal restorations.

The options for accessing a proximal lesion in a posterior tooth include approaching the lesion from the following directions:
- Occlusally, by cutting through the marginal ridge.
- Occlusally, leaving the marginal ridge intact via a tunnel preparation.
- Buccally or lingually. This is usually limited to situations where teeth are tilted lingually and where an occlusal approach would result in the removal of considerable sound tooth substance.
- Directly as a single surface, which is possible if the adjacent tooth is missing. In this case, the tooth is prepared in the same way as for the treatment of cervical or smooth surface caries.

The majority of proximal lesions are accessed from an occlusal direction, which is probably because the majority of dental schools have traditionally recommended this approach. It is helpful to consider whether it is necessary to remove the marginal ridge to access the lesion and explore whether a buccal or facial approach is possible. Tunnel approaches to access proximal lesions are technically difficult and tend to be unsuccessful in the long term, especially in premolar teeth, with fracture of the marginal ridge being a common clinical finding. Concerns have also been expressed about an operator's ability to clear the ADJ in the coronal part of the proximal preparation of caries, let alone adequately adapt the restorative material to the preparation to ensure a good tooth-restorative marginal seal – which is most important if there is some residual caries left in the preparation.

The preparations for amalgam and resin composite restorations are subtly different. However, it is still a prerequisite to break through the contact point and into the embrasure such that all contact with the adjacent tooth is removed. A common fault is not to break through the contact point. This is problematic as caries by definition is always found below the contact point.

Proximal preparations for a resin composite restoration should have a scoop form produced using a pear-shaped bur. The proximal walls are bevelled with a reciprocating handpiece or gingival margin trimmers extending the preparation just into the embrasure. Again, all friable enamel is removed but firm unsupported enamel can be left, as the restorative material will support this. No further additional preparation is required to enhance retention.

Preparations for amalgam restorations, in contrast, have a scoop-box form, which converges towards the occlusal aspect of the preparation. Again, the preparation just extends into the embrasure, although the requirement to have a certain depth (1.5 mm) of amalgam and a cavosurface margin of 90–110° makes the preparation necessarily more destructive than that required for a resincomposite restoration placed to restore a similar-sized lesion. For this reason alone, the use of amalgam in the initial operative management of an early proximal lesion that requires restoration cannot be justified. All unsupported enamel is removed, ideally with hand instruments (for example, gingival margin trimmers or alternatively safe-sided sonic preparation tips) as the use of burs to adjust proximal margins can result in damage to the adjacent tooth. If the preparation includes an occlusal lesion so that a mesio or disto-occlusal restoration is planned, further retention features are unlikely to be required. If, however, there is no occlusal lesion (i.e. a slot preparation where the marginal ridge has been removed for access to the proximal lesion), it is necessary to incorporate additional retention features in the form of retention grooves in the buccal and lingual walls of the proximal box. These grooves are prepared with a small rose-head slow-speed bur. No further preparation, other than careful finishing of the margins, is necessary.

Proximal preparations in anterior teeth
Anterior proximal lesions are universally restored with a tooth-coloured restorative material and the tooth is prepared accordingly. The lesions can be accessed:
- Labially or lingually/palatally. A lingual or palatal approach is preferable as it leaves the buccal enamel intact. If a buccal approach is indicated, it is important to minimise the buccal extent of the restoration, as the material will be susceptible to staining and discolouration. Note that unsupported buccal enamel can be left, providing it is not friable, as the restorative material will support the tooth tissue if resin-bonded. For this reason the use of resin composite is strongly recommended in anterior proximal lesions.
- Directly as a single surface, which is possible if the adjacent tooth is miss-

ing. In this case, the tooth is prepared in the same way as in the treatment of cervical or smooth surface caries.

Cervical or smooth surface preparations
These lesions only require operative intervention when attempts to arrest the lesion have failed and there is evidence of cavitation and/or lesion progression. Operative intervention is limited to accessing the lesion and extending the preparation until the ADJ is clear of caries. Caries in the deeper aspects of the preparation can then be addressed accordingly.

Managing Deep Caries

It is now accepted that in an established carious cavity softened dentine precedes discoloured dentine, which precedes infected dentine. The speed at which an individual lesion advances depends on the extent to which the effect of bacterial acids and proteases are opposed by pulpal fluid pressure, and dentine permeability. It should be noted, however, that dental caries must be within 0.5 mm of the pulp before hyperaemia and/or pulpitis will occur. It is always preferable to manage a lesion without exposing the dental pulp, possibly by using an indirect pulp-capping technique. Direct pulp-capping techniques are required when the pulp is exposed by trauma or caries. Carious exposures can be reduced by a stepwise approach to caries excavation (Fig. 3-1).

Direct pulp capping
Direct pulp capping is defined as the application of material (usually hard-setting calcium hydroxide cement) to a pulp exposed by caries or trauma. This procedure is more likely to be successful if there is no history of recurring or spontaneous pain and preoperatively there is:
• "normal" vitality
• absence of tenderness to percussion
• no radiographic evidence of periradicular pathology
• clinically a pink pulp is found, which bleeds if touched but not excessively.

The age of the pulp is also important in that younger pulps are more likely to respond positively to direct pulp-capping techniques. Biologically young pulps can be identified radiographically by an obvious pulp chamber and patent root canals. The previous restorative experience of a tooth is equally important.

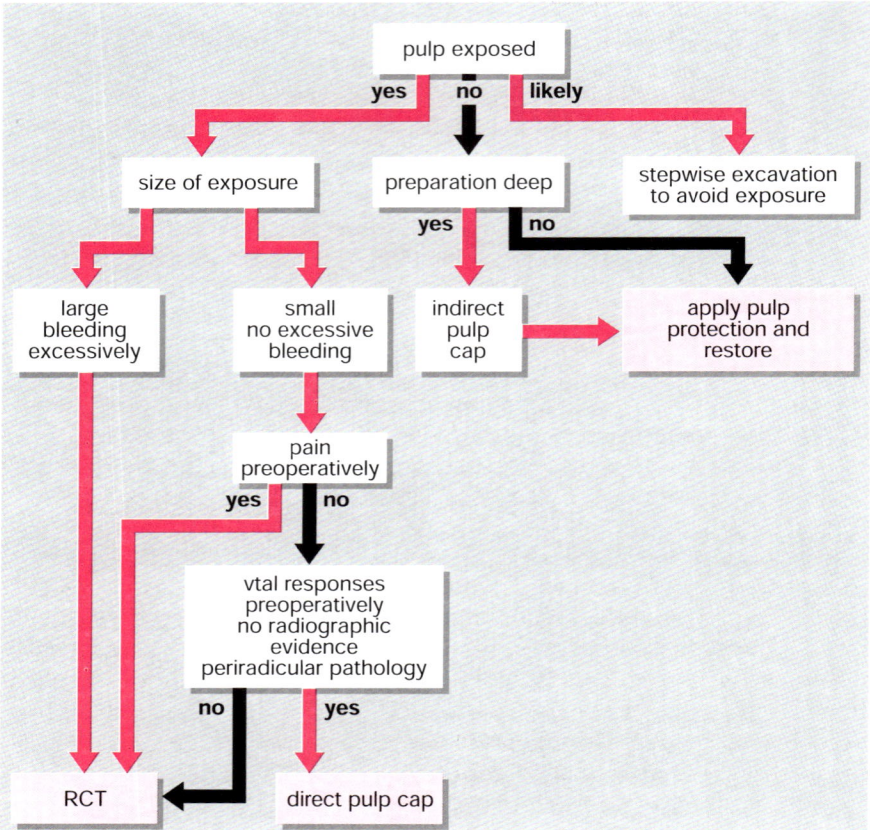

Fig 3-1 Algorithm for the management of deep caries.

Teeth with a history of pain are more likely to have bacterial invasion of the pulp and these teeth will inevitably require endodontic therapy. The position of the exposure will have an effect on the success of the procedure. The exposure should have no pulp chamber coronal to it. A cervical lesion, for example, if treated with a direct pulp cap, will heal by laying down reactionary dentine, which will interrupt the blood supply to the coronal pulp tissue leading to necrosis. If there is pulp chamber coronal to the exposure it would be sensible to consider endodontic therapy, as failure to initiate endodontics may result in a worsened prognosis due to dystrophic calcification.

The material of choice for direct pulp capping is hard-setting calcium hydroxide cement, although there is currently considerable interest in mineral trioxide aggregate (MTA) as a pulp-capping agent. It has superior therapeutic properties when compared with hard-setting calcium hydroxide cement, but it is difficult to handle and currently has a long setting reaction, which may be considered to limit its use as a pulp-capping agent.

There is little information in the literature regarding success rates for direct pulp-capping treatments. It would seem that success rates are higher for traumatic exposures than when carious exposures are treated. Further research is needed to give clearer indications as to the prognosis for pulp caps. Teeth treated in this way will always require monitoring for loss of vitality and continuing symptoms, let alone radiographic evidence of periradicular periodontitis. It is suggested that prompt endodontic therapy is indicated for teeth that have pulp caps and develop symptoms, especially if there is radiographic evidence of progressive obliteration of the root canal system.

Indirect pulp capping
Indirect pulp capping is defined as the application of therapeutic material (usually hard-setting calcium hydroxide cement) to dentine that is affected by caries but not infected with bacteria. A layer of dentine approximately 0.5 mm thick is left over the pulp and an indirect pulp-capping agent applied. It is difficult to decide when to stop excavating dentine and to determine how close to the pulp the lesion is before excavation is stopped. It has been shown that stepwise excavation results in a reduced incidence of pulpal exposure

Stepwise excavation
This is a two-stage procedure for the management of deep caries. Two visits separated by 6-12 months are required. The technique involves the following stages at the first visit:
• establishing access form
• removing superficial caries at the periphery of the preparation leaving soft, wet and pale dentine
• applying hard-setting calcium hydroxide cement to the dentine
• restoring the tooth with a traditional glass ionomer cement.
After 6-12 months, and in the absence of symptoms the second stage of the procedure involves:
• re-establishing access to the lesion
• removing the caries, which will be darker in colour, harder and drier in consistency

- indirect pulp capping with hard-setting calcium hydroxide cement and a resin-modified glass ionomer cement liner
- providing a definitive restoration.

There is considerable debate about the need to re-enter the lesion, given that the lesion is almost certainly arrested and that the tooth is frequently symptom-free. There is growing evidence that caries sealed into a tooth does not progress.

Sealing caries in
Studies have shown that caries sealed in with a fissure sealant or with resin composite does not progress because it is denied further substrate in the form of fermentable carbohydrates. The affected dentine changes to become darker, harder and drier making further operative treatment potentially unnecessary. The procedure of sealing in carious dentine will only work if a restorative material is used that seals the tooth restorative interface. Such thinking is at odds with traditional teaching in many dental schools despite the practice of sealing in dental caries compared with complete caries removal having been effectively tested in a randomised controlled clinical trial. It is suggested, therefore, that such an approach is evidence-based and is a more scientific rather than mechanistic management of dental caries. Further research is needed to evaluate the concept of sealing in dental caries.

General Points

Material selection
Before tooth preparation is started it is helpful to decide on the restorative material to be used, as this will influence the nature of the tooth preparation required. This decision may change when the extent of the lesion is determined and/or if there is fracture of undermined cusps.

Isolation
Once the outline form has been established the tooth should be isolated, ideally with rubber dam before caries removal is attempted. Rubber dam is the most effective but least used method of moisture control and tooth isolation. Practitioners seem reluctant to use rubber dam for the following reasons:
- Patients don't like it. (This is not true: patients prefer treatment under rubber dam.)
- It is difficult and time consuming to place. (This again is not true and practitioners who use rubber dam routinely become very slick at placing it.)
- The cost of the treatment is increased. (This is true, but arguably the treat-

ment is completed more rapidly, which offsets the cost of rubber dam application.)

The routine use of rubber dam is recommended because it:
• provides for better visual access
• prevents preparation contamination
• protects the airway
• reduces the risk of cross infection from patient to operator
• improves the quality of restorations significantly, particularly for the placement of resin–bonded restorations, which have been shown to have better bond strengths when placed using rubber dam because of improved moisture control.

The routine use of rubber dam is to be encouraged if we are to use more resin–bonded restorations effectively. Latex allergy is a potential difficulty that is becoming more of a problem for practitioners. Non–latex rubber dam is available and is now of comparable quality to latex dam. It is suggested, given the intimate contact of rubber dam with the soft tissues, that practitioners consider using non–latex dam routinely.

Caries removal
Caries removal is best achieved with either a slow-speed rose-head bur or excavators, although it is now accepted that manual excavation probably results in excessive removal of affected but uninfected dentine. It is preferable not to expose the pulp, so indirect pulp capping with hard-setting calcium hydroxide cement is the preferred treatment for the management of deep lesions. As a general rule, the periphery of the preparation should be cleared of caries first before the deeper areas of the preparation are managed. This is to minimise unnecessary contamination of the pulp should exposure occur during the later stages of tooth preparation.

Internal preparation features
Rounded line angles are recommended for all direct restorative materials because a rounded rather than an angular form generates less stress in the restored unit. Sharp line and point angles often require excessive removal of tooth tissue and are no longer indicated. It is helpful if replacing a failed amalgam restoration to block out any sharp line angles with a liner such as resin-modified glass-ionomer cement to produce rounded line and point angles. The curing kinetics of resin composites are significantly improved as a consequence, with reduced residual stress generated in the restored unit.

Occlusal considerations

It is vital to consider the occlusion before tooth preparation is commenced. The aim is to avoid having the tooth/restorative interface crossing occlusal contact areas. It is preferable to plan your preparation so that occlusal contact areas are on sound tooth tissue rather than the tooth–restorative interface (Figs 3-2–3-4). If this is not possible then it is legitimate to extend the preparation so that the occlusal contact area is on the restorative material rather than the tooth restorative interface.

The temptation is to under-contour restorations so that heavy occlusal loading is avoided. This will often result in movement of the opposing tooth and possible disruption to the patient's occlusal scheme. The aim is to produce a restoration that conforms to the patient's existing occlusion, including even occlusal contact in centric occlusion and immediate disclusion in lateral excursion The temptation to under-contour restorations must be resisted.

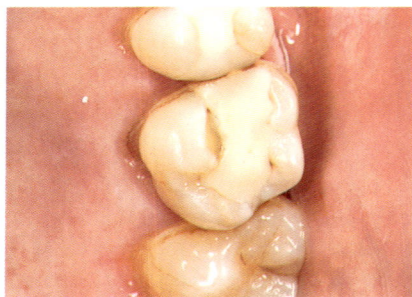

Fig 3-2 Resin-composite restoration in 26, which is over 15 years old.

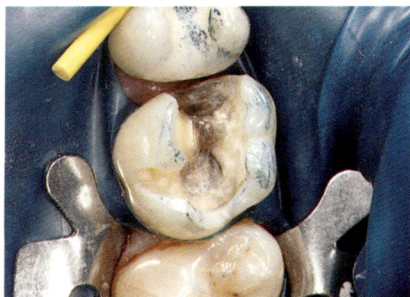

Fig 3-3 26 prepared for replacement restoration showing that the occlusion is supported by tooth tissue and not by the restorative material. This probably explains the excellent longevity for the previous restoration.

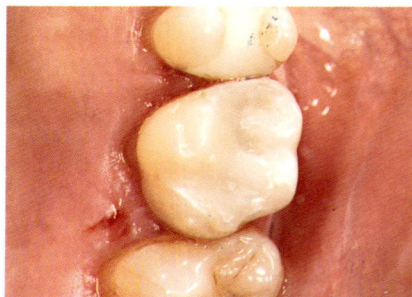

Fig 3-4 26 restored with a Giomer.

Use of magnification

There is no doubt that the use of magnification aids affords the clinician considerable advantages in operative dentistry, let alone endodontics. These include:

- clearer picture of the finer aspects of preparation form and features
- magnified view of small repairs to existing restorations (for example, repairs to the margins of crowns)
- more accurate intervention threshold whereby marginal defects are less likely to be diagnosed incorrectly as secondary caries
- better posture for the operator.

Loupes with a 2.5x magnification are the most suitable for the practice of routine operative dentistry (Fig 3-5). These can be used with an independent high-intensity attached light source. This is useful for endodontics, but the light can initiate cure of resin-based materials and is consequently, less helpful for operative dentistry. Similarly, x-ray magnifiers improve diagnosis from radiographs (Fig 3-6).

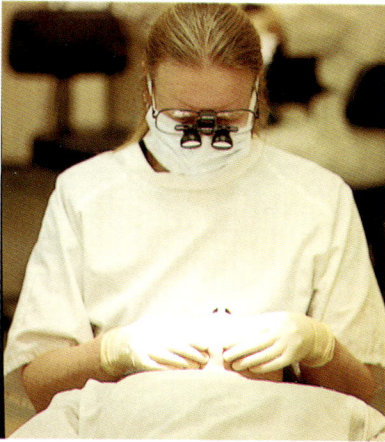

Fig 3-6 X-ray magnifier being used to view intra-oral radiographs.

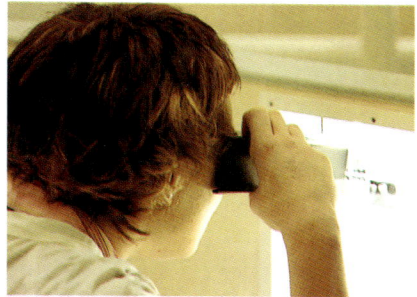

Fig 3-5 Loupes being used to examine a patient. Notice the operator's excellent posture.

Newer Preparation Techniques

Micropreparation techniques

Manufacturers of dental burs have responded to a minimally interventive approach by developing hand instruments of reduced size and, more importantly, smaller burs for micropreparation. This technique has been termed "microdentistry". The use of these burs with magnification from either a microscope or loupes allows for the very precise preparation of teeth. The burs are spherical, elliptical or tapered and allow the practitioner to explore and modify fissures even when caries has spread laterally (Figs 3-7–3-8). The burs have longer shanks, which is very helpful as the view of the bur is not obscured by the handpiece. The use of resin-bonded tooth-coloured materials in conjunction with these burs allows for a truly minimally interventive approach (Fig 3-9–3-10). The burs are designed to run at under 160,000 rpm with water coolant and therefore they can only be used in a speed-increasing handpiece (orange-ring) and not an air turbine.

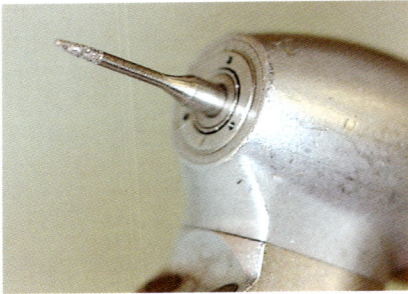

Fig 3-7 Microdentistry bur for fissure exploration.

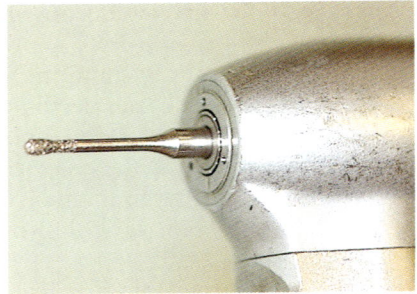

Fig 3-8 Lesion-shaped microdentistry bur.

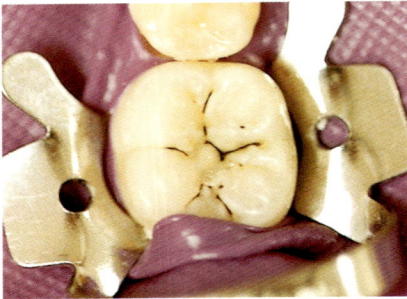

Fig 3-9 Suspicion of occlusal caries in 36.

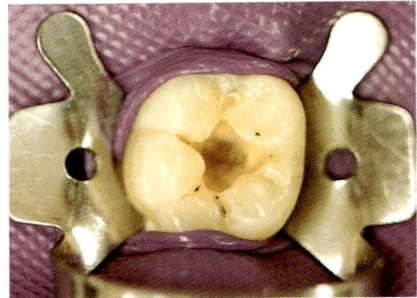

Fig 3-10 Preparation of 36 completed, with widening of the fissures prior to placement of a resin-composite restoration with fissure sealant.

Chemomechanical methods of caries removal

Chemomechanical techniques have recently been revisited and these now offer an alternative to more traditional methods of caries removal and tooth preparation. Chemomechanical caries removal involves the application of a solution to a lesion of caries, which selectively softens the carious dentine, thus facilitating its removal whilst not affecting sound non-carious dentine. This limits the removal of sound tooth structure to that required for access to the lesion.

The first commercial attempt at chemomechanical caries removal was Caridex® (National Patent Medical Products Inc.), which was initially introduced in 1985. The system involved the intermittent application of pre-heated N–monochloro–DL–2–aminobuturic acid (GK–101E) to the lesion. It was thought that the solution caused disruption of the collagen network within the lesion of caries, facilitating its removal. This method of chemomechanical caries removal was not widely adopted by practitioners, in all probability because of the expense, additional chairside time required and the bulky delivery system, which consisted of a reservoir, a heater, a pump and a handpiece with an applicator tip.

During the 1980s, a more efficient and effective chemomechanical caries removal system was developed. The material Carisolv®, which is an isotonic solution, has proved more popular with practitioners (Fig 3-11). Carisolv® contains:

- sodium hypochlorite (0.5%)
- three amino acids (glutamic acid, leusine, lysine)
- gel substance (carboxymethylcellulose)
- sodium chloride/sodium hydroxide
- saline solution
- colourant (red).

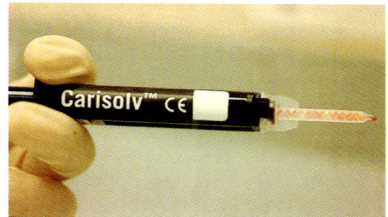

Fig 3-11 Mixed Carisolv® gel delivery system.

Chemomechanical caries removal can be used in the management of the majority of lesions, either in isolation or in conjunction with more traditional methods which may be required to gain access to the lesion and/or for the removal of existing restorations. The clinical situations in which chemomechanical caries removal could be considered the preferred method of caries removal include the treatment of:

- root/cervical caries
- coronal caries with cavitation
- caries at the margins of crowns and bridge abutments.

and

- the completion of tunnel preparations
- where local anaesthesia is contraindicated
- caries management in special needs patients and in dentally anxious patients, notably needle phobics
- atraumatic restorative technique (ART) procedures possibly provided on a domiciliary basis.

Clinical procedures
The clinical technique recommended is quickly and easily learned. It is recommended that visible and easily accessible lesions such as buccal root caries or occlusal caries with a 1–2 mm area of cavitation be attempted first. Cavitation usually helps to provide easy access for gel application and instrumentation and does not necessitate the use of a handpiece to gain access.

Specially designed hand instruments or handpieces are required. These have tips that range in diameter from 0.3 to 2 mm. These instruments may initially appear to have the look and feel of excavators, but they are designed to apply the gel and to be used in a rapid whisking or curetting fashion, which limits the removal of tooth tissue to that of carious dentine only (Fig 3-12). The different instrument configurations and tip sizes allow for access to all aspects of the lesion. The instruments also help to guide the operator around the cavity providing tactile feedback, which helps to differentiate between carious and non-carious dentine.

The effectiveness of the gel in terms of its ability to remove carious dentine effectively will begin to decrease approximately twenty to thirty minutes after mixing. Consequently, the gel should be mixed directly before use and normally be used for a single treatment only. The unmixed gel should be stored in the refrigerator, but allowed to come to room temperature prior to use.

The mixed gel is applied to the caries and left in situ for thirty seconds to allow it to start to degrade the affected dentine before the instruments are applied. Local anaesthetic is not normally required prior to the application of the gel or for caries removal. Rapid movement of the instrument coupled with light pressure facilitates caries removal. The gel must be continuously applied until cavity preparation is complete. As caries is removed, the gel becomes clouded with debris indicating that replacement gel is required and carious dentine is still present.

When cavity preparation is complete and the cavity washed and dried, the sound dentine has a slightly "frosted" and irregular appearance. This surface lacks a smear layer but has a characteristic matt finish. If kept free of contamination this surface is a good bonding substrate, particularly for fifth- and sixth-generation dentine-bonding agents. The preparation may be restored in a conventional manner, using the dental material of choice. The saucered preparation produced is ideal for restoration with a resin-bonded material.

The use of amalgam will require the preparation of undercuts.
From the patient's perspective, the response to the technique has been almost universally positive, with patients reporting less pain, discomfort and shorter perceived treatment times when compared with more conventional tooth preparation. The reduced need for the use of rotary instruments makes the experience relatively pleasant for the patient. However, in some instances, it is still necessary to use a high-speed handpiece with water coolant to gain access. A number of theories have been postulated as to why there may be reduced pain and no requirement for local anaesthesia. These include:

• Reduced cutting of caries-free dentine. Consequently, relatively few dentine tubules are exposed.

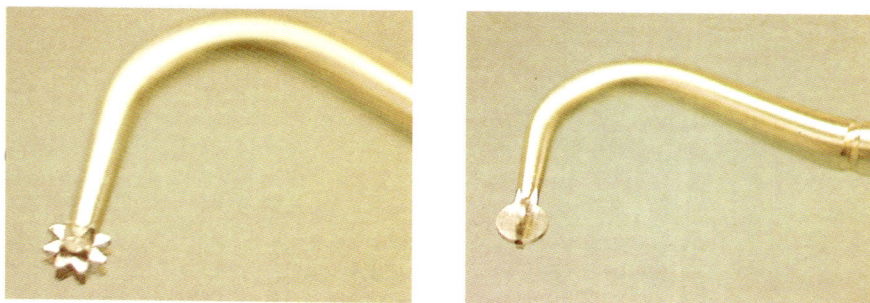

Fig 3-12 Hand instruments with special tips for chemomechanical caries removal.

- There are no vibrations from the slow-speed handpiece, no great temperature variations and the dentine is constantly covered with an isotonic gel at body temperature.
- The possible psychological input of a quiet and less traumatic experience may also play an important role. In certain cases it is necessary to administer a local anaesthetic to complete deep-cavity preparation or where existing restorations or crown and bridgework require removal prior to cavity preparation.

Although it is unlikely that chemomechanical caries removal will replace more conventional techniques, in carefully selected cases it has a place. There is little evidence to date that the outcome of treatment is different from or better than that obtained with traditional tooth–preparation techniques.

Sonic preparation
Early sonic instruments were designed for tooth preparation although they have been almost exclusively used for scaling and root surface debridement. The use of sonic preparation techniques has, however, been revisited recently. The system was initially marketed with proximal preparation tips and matched in size ceramic inserts. This type of approach is destructive of tooth tissue and has a limited application given the advantages a micro-preparation technique confers. A sonic handpiece has been developed that has three power settings, which allows for multiple applications. It has interchangeable tips, which let the practitioner carry out the following procedures:

- minimally invasive caries therapy
- preparations for indirect restorations
- luting procedures
- endodontics
- periodontics
- prophylaxis.

The handpiece works by vibration of the tips rather than rotation. It allows for precise minimal preparation of occlusal and proximal preparations. Some of the tips are coated with diamond particles on one side only and are termed "safe-sided" (Fig 3-13). These tips are very useful when proximal lesions are prepared limiting the likelihood of damaging an adjacent tooth (Figs 3-14–3-16). This allows for more flexibility in terms of how the lesion is accessed. For example, buccal or lingual access becomes a clinical possibility, which leaves the occlusal surface intact when proximal lesions are accessed. A tip has also been developed which is specifically designed to open up and extend

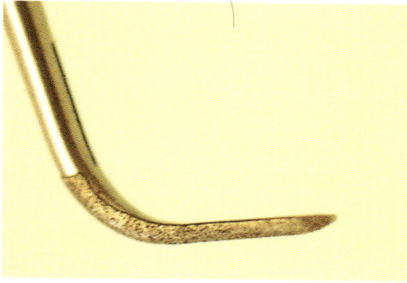

Fig 3-13 Safe-sided sonic preparation tips.

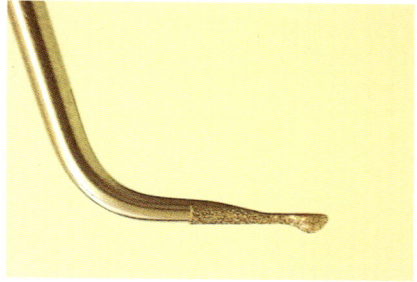

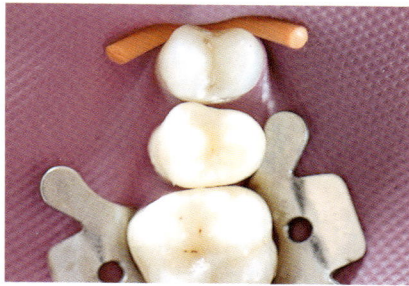

Fig 3-14 Distal lesion in 14 suitable for preparation with sonic tips.

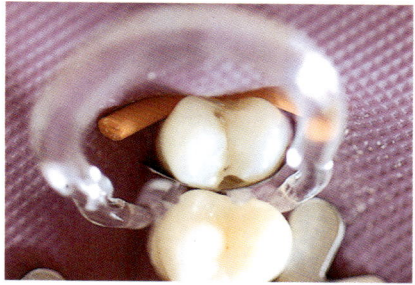

Fig 3-15 Preparation of 14 completed. A sectional matrix has been placed.

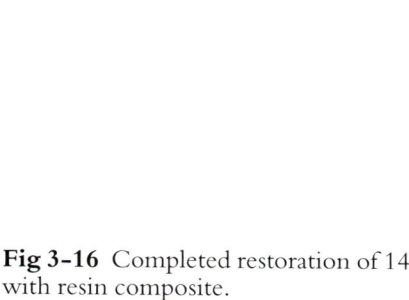

Fig 3-16 Completed restoration of 14 with resin composite.

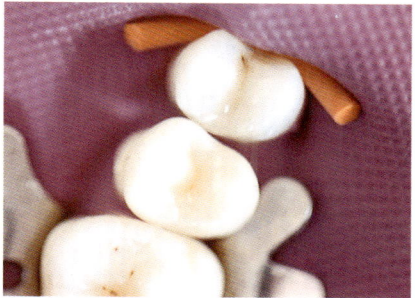

fissures as part of a sealant restoration. The tips are hard wearing, autoclavable and require replacement every nine to twelve months.

Sonic preparation, particularly with the smaller tips, is also very useful for accessing and preparing marginal defects on indirect restorations. Further research is needed to evaluate this form of tooth preparation, which could ultimately replace rotary preparation techniques in accessing and preparing small initial lesions.

Air abrasion

Air abrasion has been associated with dentistry since the 1940s. Preparation designs have changed in recent years in tandem with developments in restorative materials. Preparations with sharp line angles and undercut are not required for adhesive restorations. Consequently, air-abrasion units are enjoying a renaissance, as they are very efficient at cutting the saucer preparations recommended for adhesive restorative materials.

The units work by spraying aluminium oxide (Al_2O_3) particles (20-50μm) at a pressure of 40–140psi through a fine angled nozzle (Figs 3-17–3-18). The spray of particles cuts tooth tissue. The pressure on a standard dental unit (3–4 bar), whilst acceptable for a microetcher is insufficient for air abrasion, which requires a pressure of *c*.8 bar. Air abrasion is useful for the treatment of small initial lesions in pits and fissures and for the treatment of new caries at the margin of a restoration and in cervical areas. The system will effectively cut enamel, dentine and cementum along with restorative materials and the technique is considered to have the following advantages:

- No local anaesthesia is required for airabrasion preparation in the majority of patients. If several lesions in different quadrants require treatment in one visit this is particularly advantageous.

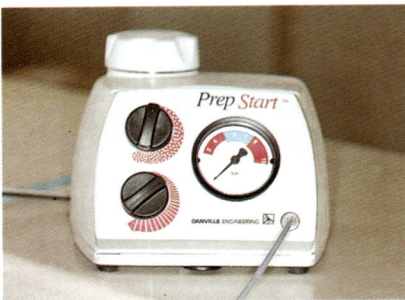

Fig 3-17 Air abrasion unit.

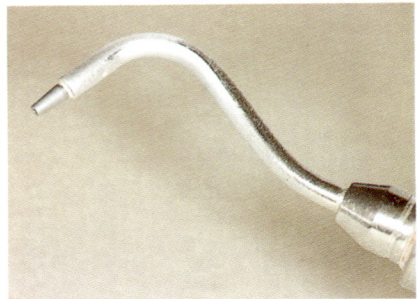

Fig 3-18 Fine nozzle of the air abrasion unit.

- The preparation produced is saucer-shaped and consequently, very preservative of tooth tissue and is eminently suitable for restoration with a resin-bonded restorative material (Figs 3-19–3-21).
- The air abrasion unit is quiet when compared with the noise of air turbines and the vibration of slow-speed handpieces.

The system does, however, have some disadvantages, which include:
- Overspray when cutting, although the newer units claim to have eliminated this problem if used with high volume suction and the unit has adequate pressure with a suitable nozzle selection. Overspray can contaminate the surgery, clog the bearings of handpieces and potentially block the filters of suction units. To overcome this problem one system uses water to reduce overspray whilst another has back suction to reduce excess dust. The dust is not considered to be dangerous but it may irritate patients who have chronic respiratory conditions such as asthma.

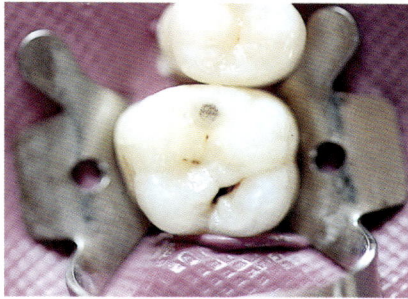

Fig 3-19 Suspicion of occlusal caries in 16.

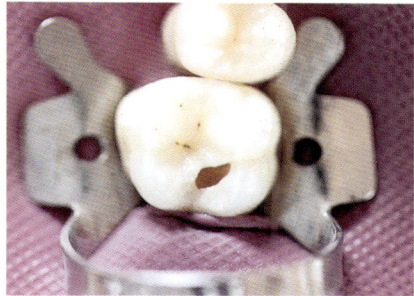

Fig 3-20 Preparation of 16 completed with air abrasion.

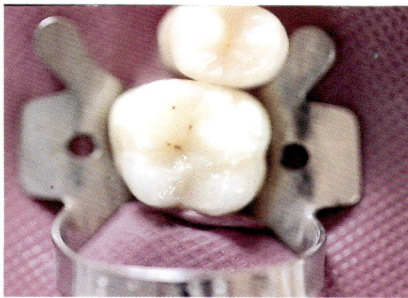

Fig 3-21 Completed restoration of 16 with resin composite.

- When proximal lesions are prepared the adjacent tooth will need protection from the overspray.
- The system is not very effective at removing soft caries and manual excavation or the use of a rose-head bur in a slow-speed handpiece is still required.
- It cannot cut precise preparations (for example, those that are required for single unit indirect restorations or fixed prosthodontic procedures).
- The systems are relatively expensive, so start-up costs are high.

If an air abrasion system is to be used the following are recommended:
- Rubber dam and protective masks to minimise patient and operator exposure to the dust.
- High-velocity suction to control overspray.
- Filter protection on the suction system to protect the pump from breakdown and the tubing from blocking.
- Abrasion-resistant or disposable mouth mirrors.
- If the air abrasion system is to be used routinely consider putting an air purification system into the surgery.

The trend to greater use of air abrasion is remarkable given the small number of studies in the literature to support its routine use. Further research is needed to provide good evidence to support the use of air abrasion at the expense of more traditional tooth preparation techniques. On a final note, air abrasion is not a substitute for acid etching and teeth prepared with aluminium oxide still require acid etching either as a separate stage or in tandem with a primer before the restorative material is placed.

Lasers
Lasers are widely used for soft tissue surgery in the UK at the present time. The lasers developed for soft tissue surgery are not suitable for hard tissue surgery and another laser system is required for hard-tissue surgery. An ideal laser system would be one that allowed both for soft and hard tissue surgery. A combined CO_2/Erbium-Yttrium Aluminium-Garnet (Er:YAG) dental laser has been developed which has such a dual application. The system allows for the cutting of enamel, dentine, bone, resin composite and soft tissue. It is reported to be as quick as a turbine, quiet, and not to require the use of local anaesthesia when enamel and dentine are prepared. These units are very expensive and whilst their use for soft tissue surgery is well documented further evaluation of their use for predictable hard-tissue surgery is needed.

Recommended Reading

Banerjee A, Watson TF, Kidd EAM. Dentine caries excavation: a review of current clinical techniques. Br Dent J 2000;188:476-482.

Kidd EAM. Caries removal and the pulpo-dentinal complex. Dent Update 2000;27:476-482.

Morrow LA Hassall DC Watts DC Wilson NHF. A chemomechanical method of caries removal. Dent Update 2000;27:398-401.

Ricketts D. Management of the deep carious lesion and the vital pulp dentine complex. Br Dent J 2001;191:606-610.

Chapter 4

Material Considerations. Which Material Today Doctor?

Aim

Practitioners are frequently uncertain as to which material to use in a given clinical situation. The aim of this chapter is to give the practitioner clear guidelines as to the situations in which dental materials can be used to both the patient's and operator's best advantage. The science behind the materials will only be discussed where it relates to the use of the material. Readers are referred to textbooks on dental materials for more detailed information.

Outcome

On reading this section practitioners will be familiar with the dental materials currently recommended for use in contemporary operative dentistry along with their respective advantages, disadvantages, indications and contraindications for use.

Introduction

There continues to be uncertainty as to which materials practitioners should use to achieve predictable results when direct restorations are being placed. This situation is not helped by materials being subject to constant change and with new materials often introduced with little information in the form of data from well-conducted clinical trials to assist practitioners in making informed decisions.

There is a move towards greater use of tooth-coloured direct restorative materials, which many believe has largely been driven by patient demand. Generally, the results achieved with these materials have been suboptimal. This is probably due to one or more of the following:
• lack of appropriate instruction
• incorrect material selection
• inappropriate clinical use – for example, using resin composite as a "white" amalgam

- not using the materials according to the directions for use especially with respect to curing depth, time of cure, application of dentine-bonding agents and with inadequate moisture control at placement
- aggressive finishing and a lack of in-service maintenance.

To assist practitioners in making appropriate decisions when selecting materials, it is helpful to review the materials currently available. The following materials and their principal advantages, disadvantages, indications and contraindications will be considered in the following section:

- amalgam
- resin composite
- compomers
- resin-modified and traditional glass ionomer cements
- ormocers
- giomers.

Common problems associated with the use of these materials and how these can best be avoided will also be addressed. It is to be remembered that no restorative material is ideal, let alone universal.

Amalgam

Introduction

Amalgam has a proven longevity with over 160 years of clinical use. Systematic reviews have claimed that amalgam has both a low cost coupled with improved longevity when compared with other materials, especially resin composite. The validity of these reviews has been questioned because the research on which these conclusions have been based relates to outdated formulations of resin composites placed using techniques that are now deprecated. Developments in the clinical application of resin composites and simultaneous developments in dentine bonding systems have shortened treatment times considerably, making the conclusions of these reviews less meaningful. Concurrently, research has also demonstrated improved longevity for resin-composite restorations above that of similar-sized amalgam restorations. There is no doubt that amalgam is a low-cost restorative material, which performs well in large preparations in premolar and permanent molar teeth, especially under occlusal loading. It is also apparent that most practitioners can readily and speedily use amalgam to good effect. Patients, however, whose needs and expectations are paramount, are increasingly dissatisfied with the continuing routine use of amalgam.

Advantages
The advantages of amalgam include:
- Ease of placement.
- Low technique sensitivity.
- Durable material with low wear rate.
- Low cost.
- Proven longevity.

Disadvantages
Amalgam has many disadvantages as a restorative material, notably:
- It is not tooth coloured.
- Undercut is required to retain the restoration (although amalgam can be bonded to teeth with dentine-bonding agents, which can reduce the need for undercuts). Bonded amalgams have proven longevities of up to two years but are much more expensive to place. It is suggested, therefore, that bonded amalgams have a place in complex or compound preparations in permanent molar teeth where the placement of dentine pins may be avoided.
- The need for undercut and to remove all unsupported enamel makes preparations for amalgam restorations necessarily more destructive of tooth tissue. Consequently, amalgam cannot be recommended for the initial management of lesions of caries and where minimal intervention is indicated.
- It is difficult to manipulate to good effect in conservative preparations.
- There is the possibility of lichenoid reactions when amalgam restorations have intimate frictional contact with adjacent mucosa – for example, cervical restorations in lower permanent molar teeth.

Indications
Amalgam is currently recommended in the following situations:
- Large compound or complex preparations in permanent molar teeth. Should additional retention be required it is preferable to bond the amalgam and/or use boxes, slots or circumferential grooves in preference to the use of dentine pins (a pin having been shown inherently to weaken the restored unit). It is likely that teeth with such extensive coronal damage are better restored with an adhesive core material rather than amalgam, followed by a full-coverage restoration such as a gold shell crown.
- Repair of fractured amalgam restorations where repair is not feasible with an adhesive material.
- As a core material – specifically as a Nayaar core in non-vital teeth – although research would seem to suggest that tooth-coloured restorative materials are equally effective in this clinical situation.

Contraindications

Current recommendations suggest that amalgam should not be used in the following situations:

- Initial lesion management where minimal operative intervention is indicated.
- In small to moderate occlusal or proximal preparations in premolar and permanent molar teeth where an adhesive material would be more appropriate (Fig 4-1).
- Large occlusal and proximal preparations in premolar teeth.
- All cervical restorations.
- For retrograde root canal therapy.
- In pregnant women.

It is suggested that the continued use of amalgam is difficult to justify in other than large preparations in posterior teeth where cusp replacement is required and a direct restoration is indicated.

Resin Composite

Introduction

These materials are a composite of glass filler particles in a resin matrix. There are many classification systems for resin composites but the system based on glass filler particle size is the most widely used. Manufacturers seem to have accepted that the concept of a universal resin composite is flawed and that resin composites for anterior and posterior use require different properties. Consequently, there is a trend away from universal resin composites.

Materials with a higher filler resin ratio are recommended for the restoration of posterior teeth whilst materials with more resin matrix at the expense of filler particles have been developed for the restoration of anterior teeth. This

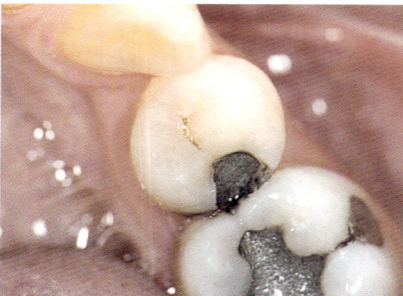

Fig 4-1 Distal aspect of 44 restored with amalgam where resin composite was indicated.

is because materials with a higher filler:resin ratio tend to be stronger, more wear resistant and shrink less when cured. A high concentration of filler particles, however, makes the materials more opaque, less vital in appearance and more difficult to polish. Conversely, materials with higher filler: resin particle ratios are more easily polished and translucent. Such materials, however, shrink more when cured.

To identify suitable materials for anterior and posterior use, practitioners are advised to look for information that relates to the percentage filler load by volume. Materials that have greater than 60% filler by volume are more suitable for the restoration of posterior teeth, whilst those below 60% filler by volume are recommended for anterior use. Manufacturers will often quote percentage filler by weight for materials, which is misleading because filler particles weigh more than the resin component. For example, a material that is 72–75% filler by weight might only be 60% filler by volume. The extent of polymerisation curing contraction is directly related to the percentage of resin in the material by volume not weight. However, several other factors are important, particularly the monomers incorporated and their specific structures and extent of cure.

Curing strategies for resin composites

Considerable research has gone into developing new resin systems with low shrinkage when cured. To date, none of this research has brought a material to the profession that has a significantly reduced polymerisation contraction when cured. It is important to recognise, therefore, that all resin systems contract on curing and that steps must be taken when placing these materials to reduce the clinical consequences of this contraction.

Currently, the majority of practitioners use a halogen bulb-based light-curing unit for photocuring resin composites. There is evidence that the maintenance of curing lights is poor, with light output in poorly maintained units being below that required: typically 400mw cm^{-2} to cure a composite adequately. Light output is reduced by debris on the light curing tip, ageing of the halogen bulb and fogging or damage to the light limiting filters. It has been shown that 25% of light-curing units have a light output below that required to cure a resin composite to an adequate depth. It is good practice therefore to check the output of the light from time to time and have the units regularly serviced (Fig 4-2). Some lights are available which can compensate for an ageing bulb. It is necessary to clean and autoclave the light-curing tip after each patient or to use a disposable sleeve.

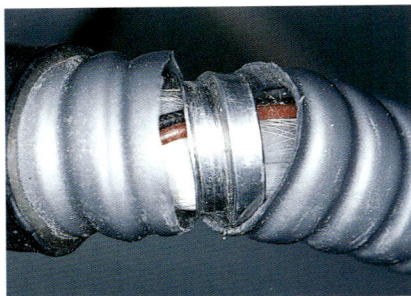

Fig 4-2 Fractured lead of halogen-based curing light still in use. A considerable proportion of the light output is lost from the lead.

A modification to the conventional light curing of resin composites was introduced recently. The concept known as "ramped" or "soft-start" polymerisation has been shown to produce better marginal adaptation, which might lead to reduced interfacial marginal leakage. It has also been suggested that the net overall shrinkage of resin composites cured with this method is less. The system works by providing a variable light output, which increases typically from 100mw cm^{-2} to 400-800mw cm^{-2} over a 40-second period (Fig 4-3). The low initial output allows for the material to reach a gel stage whereby the material can reorganise along its molecular planes accommodating initial shrinkage stress within the body of the material.

Faster curing strategies (for example, plasma-curing lights) designed to reduce shrinkage and increase depth of cure have not been demonstrated to have a significant benefit over more conventional curing strategies. Concerns have been expressed about heat generation during plasma light curing in addition to the exotherm when any resin composite polymerises, depth of cure and residual monomer post curing. It has been suggested, however, that polymerisation shrinkage is less with these lights. There is not enough evidence currently to suggest that these lights confer any advantage over a conventional halogen-based curing system, let alone a soft-start halogen-based curing light. Consequently, it is currently not possible to recommend their use.

New curing lights based on light-emitting diode (LED) technology are now available to practitioners and these look promising (Fig 4-4). The benefits of these systems are reported to be as follows:
• More energy efficient with no heat generated.
• They are quieter because no fan is needed for cooling.
• The machines are cordless, smaller and lighter.
• Depth of cure is greater than with halogen lamps.

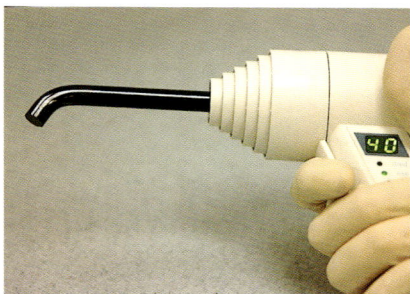

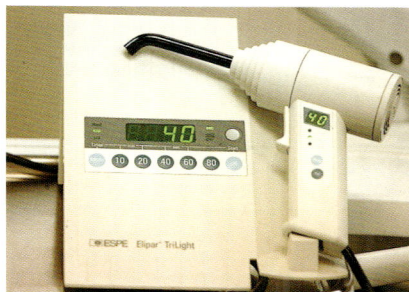

Fig 4-3 Halogen-based curing light with ramped curing mode.

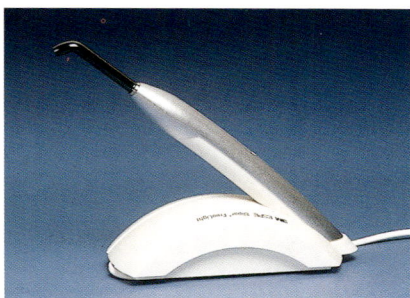

Fig 4-4 LED curing light.

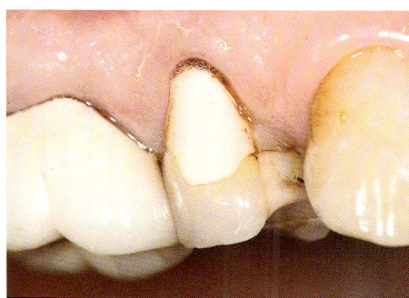

Fig 4-5 First ever light-cured resin-composite restoration placed in 15 at 25 year review.

Practitioners are advised to monitor the literature for clinical trials that support the routine use of LED lights and consider changing to these devices when the evidence suggests that an LED-based system offers some advantages over a halogen system.

Advantages

The first light-cured resin-composite restoration was placed in the UK some 25 years ago (Fig 4-5). Subsequently, manufacturers have developed many resin composite materials for use. These materials are considered to have the following advantages:

- Used in conjunction with a dentine-bonding agent they can be placed with minimal tooth preparation (Figs 4-6–4-10). In this respect these materials facilitate preservative preparation of teeth when a lesion requires operative management.

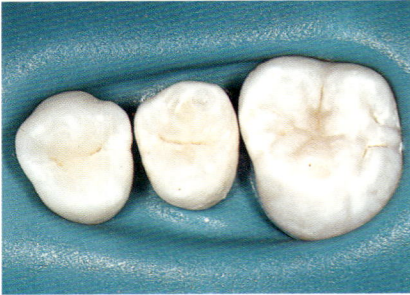

Fig 4-6 25 with distal lesion.

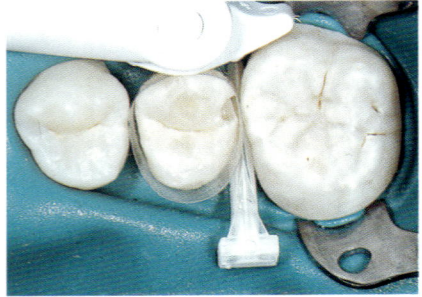

Fig 4-7 25 prepared for resin composite, disposable matrix and wedge placed.

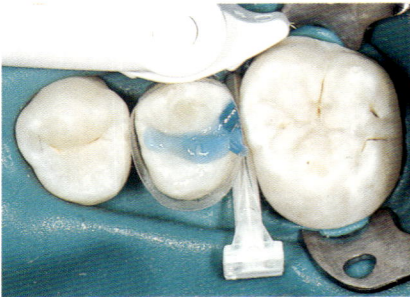

Fig 4-8 Etchant applied for 15 seconds.

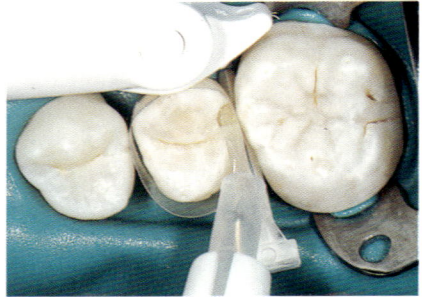

Fig 4-9 Application of fifth-generation dentine-bonding agent.

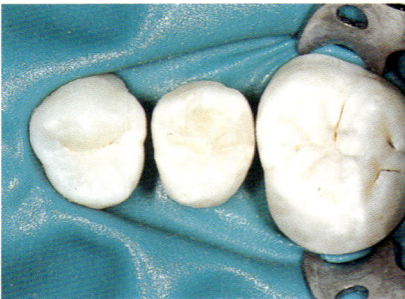

Fig 4-10 Completed restoration of 25 with resin composite.

- Light curing allows for command cure, which allows for immediate finishing and polishing.
- The restoration, if placed correctly in suitably selected teeth, seals the tooth restorative interface, reducing interfacial leakage.
- It is possible to add material to cured increments, which allows for incremental build-up and further additions at a later date, which makes resin-composite restorations repairable.
- They are tooth coloured.
- Single-paste systems have good handling and limited porosity.

Disadvantages
Resin composite materials suffer certain limitations, which include the following:
- The chemistry (i.e. the conversion from monomer to polymer when the material is light, or chemically, cured) results in material shrinkage of 2–3%. This can disrupt the marginal adaptation of the material, fracture weakened cusps and produce post-operative sensitivity leading to early failure of the restoration in clinical service.
- Bonding to dentine still remains problematic, especially at the margins of a preparation (for example, the floor of the box when the floor is below the cemento-enamel junction (CEJ) in proximal preparations).
- The replacement of missing cusps in large preparations in posterior teeth, although thought to be inappropriate with resin composites placed directly, this has not been tested in a clinical trial.
- Water absorption with surface and marginal staining after some years of clinical service.
- Patient and operator sensitivity to the components of bonding resins, in particular HEMA.

Indications
Current indications for resin composites include:
- Small, medium and large occlusal restorations in posterior teeth.
- Small, medium and large proximal restorations in premolar teeth and small to medium proximal preparations in permanent molar teeth. Where the proximal margins are below the CEJ, a bonded-base approach is indicated.
- Cervical lesions in all teeth.
- Incisal edge restorations.
- Diagnostic build-up and definitive restorations in tooth wear cases.
- Canine risers.
- Fissure sealants.

Contraindications
It is suggested that resin composite should not be used in the following situations:
- Large proximal preparations where cusps require replacement in permanent molar teeth.
- Where it is not possible effectively to isolate the operative field (for example, DO preparations in third molars).
- Restoration of root caries.
- Where patients have a proven allergy to one or more of the constituents of the resin-based restorative systems.

Flowable resin composites
Flowable resin composites were introduced to practitioners relatively recently. These materials are characterised by having a lower filler:resin ratio. Consequently, these materials will suffer relatively large percentage shrinkage when they are cured but have the advantage of ease of adaptation to preparations. They are useful for and indicated in the following situations:
- Repair of marginal defects in restorations.
- As a liner, especially to block out undercuts.
- As the initial increment on the cervical floor of proximal preparations where the preparation is above the CEJ. The use of a resin-modified glass ionomer cement is recommended when the preparation extends below the CEJ.

Tips for using resin composites
Resin composites are technique sensitive. However, the results achieved are generally excellent in carefully selected cases. Success is more likely if attention is paid to the following:
- Do not attempt to pack or condense the resin composite. They are not "white" amalgam and should be handled differently. Resin composite should be adapted and contoured to the preparation. Packing of resin-based products, particularly with a poorly adapted matrix band, is associated with an increased incidence of overhang formation that is often difficult to remove.
- In proximal preparations it is advantageous to build up the marginal ridge of the restoration in the first instance. Further build-up can be as for an occlusal preparation, which simplifies the process.
- Try not to connect two opposing walls when an increment is placed as it puts the opposing walls under stress when the increment is cured. A clinical example of this is bulk curing of a large mesio-occlusal-distal resin composite placed in premolar teeth where a crack is noted at the base of

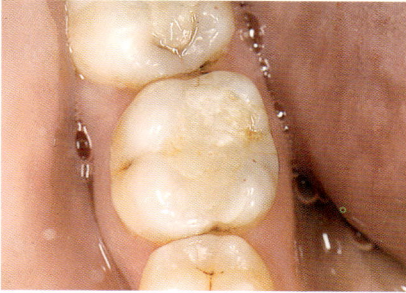

Fig 4-11 Bulk cure of occlusal resin composite in 46 resulting in fracture of the disto-lingual cusp.

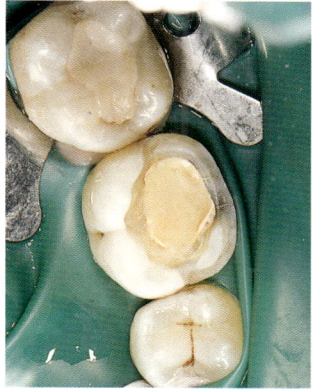

Fig 4-12 Preparation of 46 for indirect resin composite inlay after amputation of the fractured disto-lingual cusp.

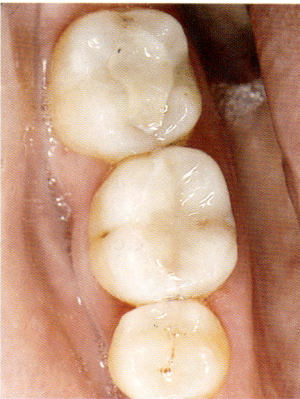

Fig 4-13 Cemented inlay in 46.

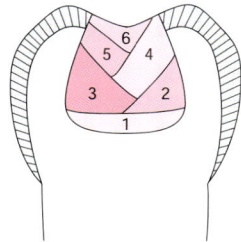

Fig 4-14 Incremental build-up technique.

a cusp post curing (Figs 4-11–4-13). Oblique increments are recommended for this reason (Fig 4-14).

- Do not use transparent matrix bands as they confer no advantage, and apart from the difficulty of using them they are so thick they may under-contour the contact point. Metal bands have been shown to be equally effective for the placement of proximal resin composites, provided additional trans-tooth curing is done in the form of 20-second curing from either side of the embrasure after the band is removed. The use of metal bands allows for better contact formation and permits wooden wedges to

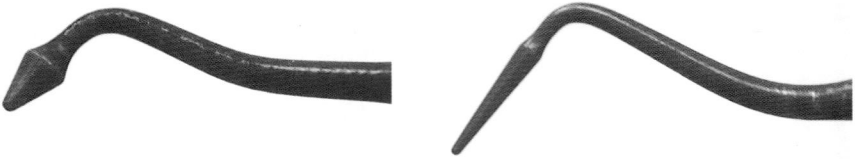

Fig 4-15 Instrument tips designed specifically for the manipulation of resin composite.

be used. Sectional matrices are especially useful for forming contact points in proximal resin-composite restorations (Fig 3-15).
- Use separate instruments for resin composite. Several manufacturers market non-stick instruments specially for resin-based restorative materials (Fig 4-15).
- The curing of resin composite is inhibited by oxygen, which is helpful in that each cured increment has uncured monomer on the surface to which additional increments can be added. This is undesirable for the final increment placed and for that reason it is preferable to overbuild the restoration and cut it back during finishing and polishing. An alternative would be to contour the final increment anatomically and then apply airblock, which excludes oxygen before curing.
- The use of a wedge is important when proximal preparations are restored. It creates a potential space for the interdental papillae and allows for tight contact point formation especially when resin composite restorations are placed. Do not simultaneously wedge the tooth mesially and distally, as this will extrude the tooth. Consequently, the restoration will be over-contoured when the occlusion is checked to accommodate the occlusion. If mesial and distal preparations are to be restored together, wedge either mesially or distally first, place the restorative material and then move the wedge to the other preparation.

Dentine-bonding agents
In recent years there have been rapid developments in the chemistry of dentine-bonding agents. In tandem, our understanding of how dentine-bonding agents work and how they should be applied to maximum benefit has developed. It is now possible reliably to bond to dentine through cohesive hybridisation of dentine. Essentially, dentine-bonding agents contain three components:

- an etchant or conditioner, which is either 37% ortho phosphoric acid or a weak organic acid
- a primer such as HEMA with a diluent monomer such as TEGMA
- a bonding resin typically based on Bis-GMA.

Currently, sixth-generation dentine-bonding agents are available combining all these components in one product, which requires multiple applications. Fifth-generation bonding agents have a separate etch stage followed by simultaneous application of a combined primer and bonding resin, which usually require two applications. Alternatively, the primer is combined with the etchant followed by subsequent application of a bonding resin. Fourth-generation bonding agents have three distinct stages (etchant, primer and bonding agent).

The fourth-generation three-bottle systems are arguably the gold standard against which newer systems are compared and tested. It is accepted that the best results are achieved with three-bottle systems. Fifth-generation systems are relatively tried and tested and give good clinical results if the directions for use are followed. The sixth-generation systems are in their infancy. The results are good on enamel but less certain when dentine is treated. Doubtless these systems will improve and practitioners are advised to monitor the literature for clinical trials demonstrating significant advantages for these systems over more proven ones.

Wet bonding

For successful cohesive hybridisation of dentine with a resin system, conditioned dentine should be left moist. Excessive dehydration of dentine will result in collapse of the collagen framework and produce lower bond strengths when resin is applied. Practitioners struggle with this concept and there is great variability in how much residual moisture is and should be left in the dentine. One advantage of a sixth-generation system is that this variable is removed, as no drying of dentine is required.

Tips for using bonding agents

To maximise the results achieved with a bonding system it is recommended that careful attention is paid to the following:

- Follow the manufacturer's directions for use.
- Use a bonding system and resin composite from the same manufacturer, as the resin chemistry will be compatible.
- Do not over-etch dentine. Treatment times in excess of 15 seconds will result in post-operative hypersensitivity due to nanoleakage. Nanoleakage

occurs when resin uptake is less than the depth of the etchant penetration, leaving a gap.

- Apply dentine-bonding agents to proximal preparations before the matrix band is applied so that the cervical margin is adequately treated prior to the application of the first increment of resin composite.
- Whilst it is important to evaporate the solvent from the dentine-bonding agent, it is critical that this process is gradual. Aggressive use of a three-in-one syringe will thin the resin layer and result in poor film thickness, remembering that the resin's secondary function is to seal the dentine.
- When the restoration is finished, apply a further layer of bonding resin to act as a surface treatment. Surface treatment resin penetrates surface cracks and strengthens the surface layer.

Compomers

Introduction

Compomers were introduced into the UK in 1993 and are essentially a form of resin composites in another guise. The material is made predominately from resin composite (*c*.90%) with the addition of a polyacid-modified molecule similar to that found in traditional glass ionomer cement. Compomers are initially light cured but subsequently absorb water, allowing for an acid-based reaction to set the polyacid-modified molecule. Consequently, the material shrinks – initially due to polymerisation contraction – and expands subsequently as water is absorbed. The net expansion, however, is never as much as the initial shrinkage. The addition of the polyacid-modified molecule makes the material more hydrophilic. It is, therefore, relatively easy to handle and adapt to preparations, which possibly explains why this group of materials is so popular with practitioners. The dominance of these materials by resin composite means that they are resin based and a dentine-bonding agent is required for their successful placement. Physically, the properties of these materials are similar to those of resin composite. However, wear rates and fracture resistance are, for example, less than those for resin composite.

Advantages

Compomers and resin composites share the same advantages. Additional advantages include fluoride release and ease of handling. Manufacturers have suggested from time to time that these materials can be placed without the use of a dentine-bonding agent, which is difficult to reconcile with the material's chemistry. It is recommended, therefore, that if a compomer is used, a dentine-bonding agent be used as well.

Disadvantages
These are similar to the disadvantages of resin composites.

Indications
There are no clear indications for the use of compomers. Indeed, it is difficult to identify an indication for compomer where the use of a compomer would confer an advantage over the use of a resin composite. Consequently, it has been argued that they are a redundant class of materials.

The only situation where the use of a more hydrophilic resin system (i.e. a compomer) might be advantageous is in the restoration of non-carious and carious cervical lesions where moisture control can be problematical. The hydrophilic nature does not mean that the material can tolerate excess moisture in the form of saliva, and as with all resin-bonded restorations the use of a rubber dam during the placement of these materials is strongly recommended. The modulus of elasticity of compomers is lower than resin composite and the material is less rigid as a consequence. This might confer some advantage in non-carious cervical lesions if tooth flexure is responsible for the lesion. The rigidity of resin composite might explain the poor retention rates recorded for restorations of such materials. Further research is indicated to determine if compomer restorations have increased retention rates in this clinical situation.

Contraindications
These again are similar to those for resin composite.

Resin-modified and Traditional Glass Ionomer Cements

Introduction
Glass ionomers were developed in the UK and have been used extensively for over twenty years, notably in the UK and Australasia. Generically, the materials are similar with resin-modified glass ionomer cements, differing only from traditional glass ionomer cements in that 20% of the material comprises a resin-based material. These materials are aqueous based rather than resin based and do not require the use of a dentine-bonding agent. Superior results will be achieved with these materials if a tooth conditioner in the form of a weak organic acid is used prior to application. A tooth conditioner is often supplied with the material but practitioners seem reluctant to use them.

Advantages
These materials have the following advantages:
• They develop self-adhesion to tooth tissue through bioreacting with the

tooth surface. This process is enhanced if the tooth surface is conditioned and left moist prior to application of the material.

- The resin-based systems are command cured although it is important to understand that the acid-base reaction for the traditional glass ionomer cement proportion of the material (c.80%) is really how the material cures and sets. This reaction is dependent on water absorption and takes several days for the process to be complete. More correctly, therefore, resin-modified glass ionomer cements are initially photo-stabilised rather than light cured.
- The materials are tooth-coloured.
- Fluoride release.

Disadvantages

The materials have disadvantages linked to their inferior physical properties when compared with resin composites. These disadvantages include:

- Poor fracture strength and wear rates.
- Water absorption in resin-modified glass ionomer cements makes them unsuitable for use as luting cements for all ceramic restorations, as there is a net expansion of 4% which places all ceramic restorations under undue stress.
- Marginal chipping of traditional glass ionomer cements, particularly when they have been used to restore occlusal preparations.
- Traditional glass ionomer cements tend to be more opaque and less aesthetic than resin-modified glass ionomer cements.
- Exogenous stain build-up is common with traditional glass ionomer cements.

Indications

Glass ionomer cements are indicated for use in the following circumstances:

- Liners and bases for direct and indirect restorations.
- Resin-modified glass ionomer cements are indicated for bonded-base restorations.
- Temporary restorations, especially between appointments in endodontic therapy.
- Transitional restorations for rapid stabilisation of a dentition where there are multiple cavities in a patient with a high caries risk.
- Atraumatic Restorative Technique (ART).
- Cementation of cast indirect restorations.
- Traditional glass ionomer cements are useful for the restoration of root caries in the elderly patient.

Contraindications

Glass ionomer cements are not indicated in the following situations:

- Definitive restorations in the adult dentition except for the treatment of root caries.
- Resin-modified glass ionomer luting cements are not suitable for luting of all-ceramic restorations as they expand due to water absorption, the expansive force of which can result in fracture of the restoration.

Ormocers

These materials are organically modified ceramics, also known as organically modified silicates. Their chemistry is based on a polyvinylsiloxane backbone. Several materials have been introduced, but there is very little evidence to support their use, as there is some doubt as to what advantage these materials have over amalgam and resin composite.

Giomers

This is a new group of materials released in the UK very recently. The material unites the chemistries of resin composite and glass ionomer in an effort to combine the advantages of both materials whilst minimizing the limitations of each. The material is composed of pre-reacted glass ionomer particles within a resin matrix. Giomers can be subdivided into two distinct groups of materials – namely, those where the glass ionomer particles have surface reacted and those which have fully reacted. Surface pre-reacted glass ionomer giomers (S-PRG) are suitable for resin composite indications, whilst fully pre-reacted glass ionomer giomers (F-PRG) are used in a dentine-bonding agent, fissure sealant and as a restorative material for non-load-bearing areas. This group of materials are used with a fifth-generation dentine-bonding agent, which has a conditioning primer and a bonding agent that is enriched with fluoride. Three-year results of a multi-centre clinical trial of a S-PRG restorative material have demonstrated its suitability for occlusal and proximal preparations in posterior teeth.

A remarkable feature of this group of materials is their proven ability to release fluoride and to recharge by absorbing fluoride. It has been suggested that the material discharges fluoride when intra-oral fluoride levels are low and recharges when intra-oral fluoride levels are high. Although the therapeutic benefits of this fluoride interaction have yet to be demonstrated clinically, and the benefits of fluoride release are currently being questioned, this is still a novel property of this group of materials. The F-PRG group of giomers absorbs significant amounts of water once cured. This may have a clinical consequence and currently clinical trials of this group of materials are ongoing prior to release of the material for clinical use. Currently, F-PRG giomers are limited to use in a dentine-bonding agent.

General Points

Fluoride release
There is a great deal of debate in the literature concerning fluoride release from restorative materials. A recent systematic review has demonstrated that research, to date, has failed to demonstrate a therapeutic benefit associated with fluoride release from a dental material. If fluoride release is to be beneficial then it must be sustained and the material should be rechargeable by

Table 4-1 Summary of different material indications.

Amalgam	• large complex/compound preparation in molar teeth • repair of amalgam restorations
Resin composite	• occlusal and proximal restorations in posterior teeth except large restorations in molar teeth • anterior proximal restorations • cervical restorations • incisal edge restorations • canine risers • fissure sealants
Compomers	• non-carious cervical lesions
Resin-modified glass ionomer cements	• liners • bases • temporary/diagnostic restorations • ART • luting cements
Traditional glass ionomer cements	• treatment of root caries

fluoride toothpaste/gel and or a mouthwash. As a general note, manufacturers tend to report cumulative fluoride release rather than sustained fluoride release. Until such time as there is robust evidence to suggest fluoride release is beneficial, practitioners should not give undue weight to manufacturers' claims of fluoride release when selecting a material.

Antimicrobial release

This is an area that merits exploration in the future. It has been shown that chlorhexidine can reduce caries risk, and patients on a preventive regime that includes chlorhexidine develop fewer lesions of caries. Toothpastes that contain Triclosan work in a similar way and already there is a resin system that contains Triclosan on the market. The material is for sealing and protecting exposed root surfaces. Triclosan is included to reduce the risk of future root caries. More clinical trials are needed in this area.

Conclusions

In the next few years it is likely that resin composites will replace amalgam as the primary restorative material for the direct restoration of the adult dentition (Table 4-1). Currently, the use of amalgam for the initial management of carious cavities cannot be justified. Glass ionomer cements, whether resin-modified or not, should be used for liners and/or bases and for the management of root caries only. The literature should be monitored to see if ormocers and giomers are demonstrated to have proven advantages over resin composite. Successful manipulation and use of dental materials is operator specific and practitioners are recommended to use a few materials frequently and only change from materials that work well when the evidence suggests the newer material has a proven advantage.

Recommended Reading

Hickel R, Dasch W, Janda R, Tyas M, Anusavice K. New direct restorative materials. Int Dent J 1998:48;3-16.

Chapter 5
Pulp Protection Regimes. Sealers, Liners and Bases

Aim

Pulp protection regimes have changed dramatically over recent years. The aim of this chapter is to update the practitioner about contemporary pulp protection regimes.

Outcome

At the end of this section practitioners will be familiar with modern pulp protection regimes and recognise the clinical indications for sealers, liners and bases.

Introduction

Bacterial contamination of dentinal tubules and subsequently the pulp is the principal cause of pulpal inflammation. The direct toxic effects on the pulp of restorative materials have been shown to be mild and transitory. The pulp may have been inflamed prior to a restoration being placed but this inflammation will largely resolve following treatment (reversible pulpitis) provided further bacterial contamination is prevented. The pulp may also be damaged due to sudden and excessive rises in temperature generated during the restorative procedure through inadequate water-cooling of burs, use of worn burs and/or inadequately maintained handpieces and excessive dehydration of the pulp during operative procedures. It is important, therefore, to maintain handpieces with regular servicing and to replace burs which have become worn. Single-use burs offer obvious advantages in this respect.

Accidental entry into the pulp chamber (pulpal exposure) by a hand or rotary instrument (traumatic exposure) will damage the pulp. Accurate knowledge of the anatomy of each tooth is therefore essential to ensure that tooth preparation is completed with the minimum of iatrogenic damage. An important consideration is the age of the patient, as younger patients have larger pulp chambers than older patients. Previous restorative treatment and other insults to the pulp will have resulted in a reduction in the size of the pulp chamber due to secondary dentine being laid down.

To prevent noxious stimuli reaching the pulp it has been custom and practice to apply protective materials to the floor and/or the pulpo-axial wall of preparations. These materials were commonly placed under amalgams and resin composites to prevent thermal stimulation of the pulp and acid contamination of dentine respectively. It has been demonstrated that thermal stimulation of dentine is not normally a problem clinically and that routine basing of preparations for amalgams, to prevent thermal stimulation, inherently weakens the restoration without benefit to the continuing vitality of the tooth. It is also accepted that dentine can be etched without deleterious pulpal effects and therefore routine lining of preparations for resin composites is now contraindicated.

It is currently suggested that the routine placement of a preparation liner or base is contraindicated. All preparations should, however, have some form of sealer applied and some preparations (usually deep) will require a liner and/or base (Fig 5-1). There is some merit in etching preparations prior to placing a sealer, liner or base, as etching will remove the smear layer, which is contaminated with bacteria. Removal of the smear layer in this way affords gross debridement of the preparation and will also improve the quality of the interface between the sealer/liner and the dentine substrate.

Sealers
A preparation sealer is a material which seals the dentinal tubules and provides a protective coating for freshly cut dentine. Examples of sealers include copal ether cavity varnish and dentine desensitisers.

Liners
Preparation liners also seal freshly cut dentine but have additional functions such as adhesion to tooth structure, fluoride release, and/or antibacterial action. Preparation liners are applied in thin section (>0.5 mm), and materials currently used include resin-modified glass ionomer cements, dentine-bonding agents, flowable resin composites and hard-setting calcium hydroxide cements. It has been suggested that resin-modified glass ionomer cements have greater resistance to microleakage than dentine-bonding agents. This feature can be used to good advantage when planning to place an amalgam in a deep preparation.

amalgam preparations

minimal	deep	very deep

| (S) with dentine desensitiser | (S) and (L) with resin-modified glass ionomer cement | (S) and (L) with resin-modified glass ionomer cement always and hard-setting calcium hydroxide cement in deeper areas if indicated |

In complex or compound amalgams a dentine-bonding agent should be used

resin composite preparations

minimal	deep	very deep

| (S) with dentine bonding agent | (S) with dentine bonding agent | (L) with hard-setting calcium hydroxide cement in deeper areas if indicated and (S) with a dentine bonding agent |

Remember that dentine-bonding agents primarily have a bonding function as well

Definitions

Term	Definition
S	Sealer
L	Liner
B	Base
Minimal preparation	just in to dentine
Deep preparation	only 2 mm of dentine remaining
Very deep preparation	less than 2 mm dentine remaining

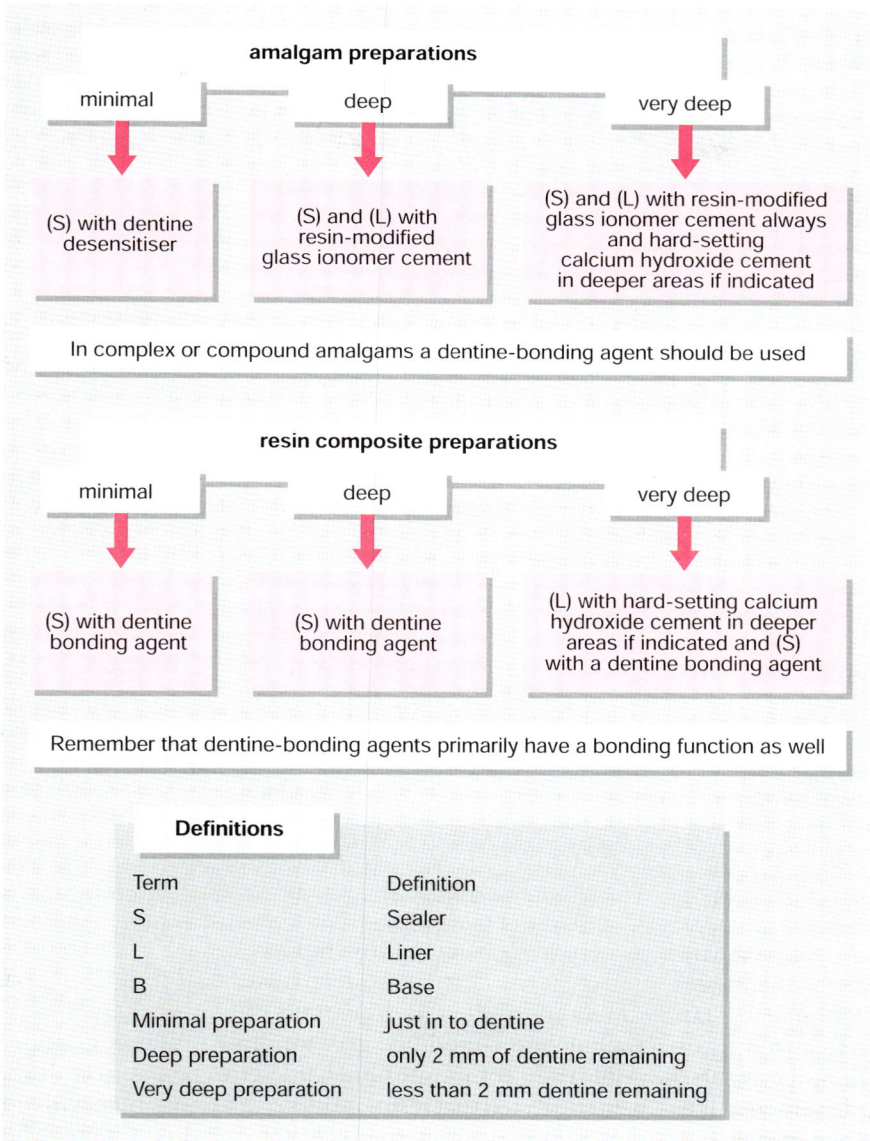

Fig 5-1 Algorithm for pulp-protection regimes.

It has been recommended that the resin-modified glass ionomer cement liner should be applied to the preparation and not cured with the amalgam packed directly onto the liner. The rationale behind this approach is that the liner will chemically cure whilst developing adhesion both to the tooth and the amalgam restoration, further enhancing restoration retention. Some clinicians advocate that two layers of resin-modified glass ionomer cement should be applied in this approach, with only the first layer being cured. To date, there is no evidence in the form of well-conducted clinical trials to demonstrate the benefit to lining amalgam preparations in this way.

If a dentine-bonding agent is used it is recommended that a filled resin system (i.e. one that contains filler particles) should be used as it is easier for the operator to ensure that all dentine is covered, sealed and lined. The thickness of the layer is important in that it provides an elastic interface between the tooth and the restorative material, which allows for relief of stresses generated by curing contraction.

There is continuing controversy regarding the use of different hard-setting calcium hydroxide cement preparations for direct and indirect pulp capping. Similarly, the wisdom of etching pulpal tissue, let alone the direct application of dentine-bonding agents to the dental pulp, is controversial. Currently, there is no evidence to support the etching and direct application of bonding agents to pulpal tissue. Research has shown that residual monomer found in the pulp chamber is associated with inflammation and poor calcific repair. There is also the possibility of sensitising the patient to components of the resin system, notably HEMA.

Bases

Bases are dentine replacements, which reduce the bulk of directly placed restorative material – for example, amalgam. They are also used to block out preparation undercuts when indirect restorations are prescribed. Traditional and resin-modified glass ionomer cements are examples of bases. Historically, zinc oxide-eugenol and zinc phosphate have also been used as bases. It is difficult, however, to recommend their continued use given the superior properties of traditional and resin-modified glass ionomer cements. The routine basing of restorations to prevent thermal shocking of the pulp through metallic restorations is contraindicated, as thermal stimulation of the pulp through metallic restorations has not been shown to be problematical.

Bonded bases

Bases are traditionally confined to the preparation and are not exposed to the oral environment. Proximal resin-composite restorations are problematic when the cervical floor of the preparation is below the CEJ. In an effort to improve marginal adaptation and reduce cervical gap formation, open-sandwich-type restorations were described in which traditional glass ionomer cements were used in thin section on the cervical floor of proximal preparations to improve marginal adaptation. Unfortunately, the longevity of these restorations was poor, with the glass ionomer cement prone to washout with subsequent collapse of the restoration. Recently, this technique has been modified to include the use of resin-modified glass ionomer cements in open-sandwich-type restorations. These restorations have improved longevity, with survival rates of up to seven years reported (Figs 5-2–5-8).

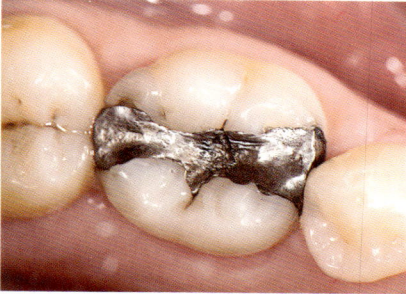

Fig 5-2 Failed MOD amalgam restoration in 36.

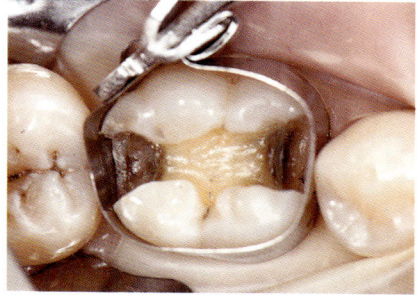

Fig 5-3 Restoration removed from 36 reveals boxes are below the CEJ.

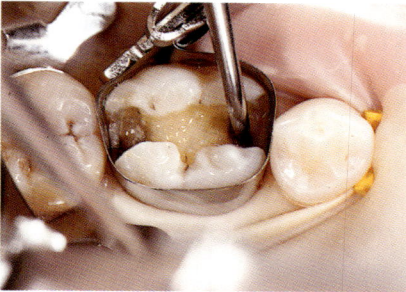

Fig 5-4 Placement of 1mm increment of resin-modified glass ionomer cement.

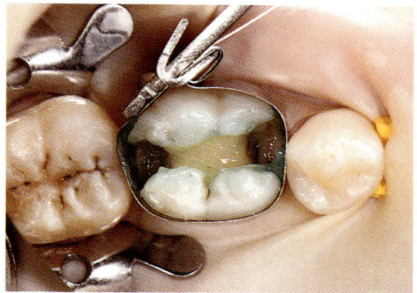

Fig 5-5 Etchant placed for 15 seconds.

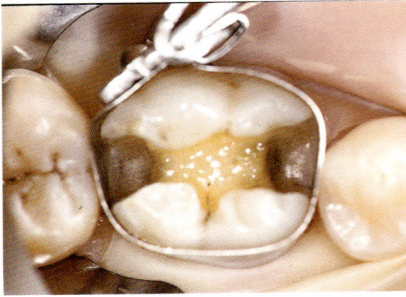

Fig 5-6 Preparation after removal of etchant.

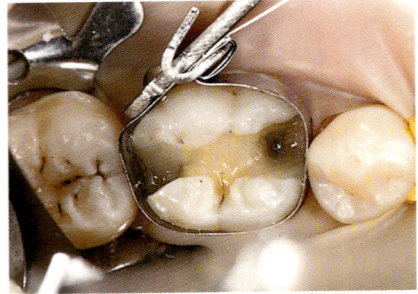

Fig 5-7 Placement of oblique increments of resin composite.

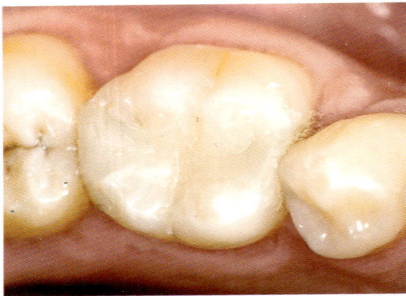

Fig 5-8 Finished resin-composite restoration in 36.

Indications for Sealers, Liners and Bases

Amalgam restorations

Dentine itself is an excellent insulator. In preparations with more than 2 mm of remaining dentine thickness, therefore, there is generally no requirement for any pulp protective material other than a preparation sealer prior to restoration placement. The thickness of the dentine is assessed using radiographs and the clinician's knowledge of tooth anatomy weighed against the age of the patient and previous restorative therapy. A preparation sealer will seal dentinal tubules and prevent both post-operative sensitivity and bacterial recontamination of dentinal tubules. In the case of simple amalgam restorations, two coats of a dentine desensitiser are recommended. Current indications would seem to suggest that dentine desensitisers have largely replaced cavity varnish as a preparation sealer for amalgam restorations and it is difficult to justify the continued use of cavity vanish. There is insufficient evidence at present, however, to support the routine use of dentine-bonding agents under amalgam restorations. There is growing evidence, however, that compound complex amalgams would benefit from the application of a dentine-bonding agent or resin-luting cement, which has a special affinity for metal. The bonding of amalgam restorations in this way, together with techniques to maximise resistance and retention form in preparations, has, in the opinion of many practitioners, made dentine pins, with all their inherent disadvantages, redundant.

For deeper cavities, where there is less than 2 mm of remaining dentine, a preparation liner should be placed in the deepest aspects of the preparation. It is usual to place a small increment of hard-setting calcium hydroxide cement in the deepest aspects, but only if a pulp exposure is evident or a micro exposure suspected, and then place resin-modified glass ionomer cement over all remaining dentine. This is termed direct pulp capping. In very deep cavities in which the pulp is nearly exposed, hard-setting calcium hydroxide cement is applied to this area only and then a resin-modified glass ionomer cement liner is placed. This is termed "indirect pulp capping". It is important to minimise the extent and thickness of the hard-setting calcium hydroxide cement, as the material is weak and prone to fracture under restorations.

There continues to be debate in the literature regarding the use of hard-setting calcium hydroxide cement. At present, however, the evidence supports its minimal use as a direct and indirect pulp-capping agent. If hard-setting calcium hydroxide cement is used it is not possible to use a sixth-generation dentine-bonding agent. The acidic primers have a low pH, which will dissolve the hard-setting calcium hydroxide cement. To prevent this, cover the hard-setting calcium hydroxide cement with resin-modified glass ionomer cement.

Resin-composite restorations
Dentine-bonding agents should be routinely used under all resin-composite restorations. Dentine-bonding agents primarily retain the restoration but have another function – namely, that of sealing the dentinal tubules, preventing post-operative sensitivity and bacterial contamination of the tubules. It is important that when dentine-bonding agents are applied that all dentine surfaces of the preparation are covered by a sufficient thickness of the agent. Multiple applications are often required along with prudent use of the 3-in-1 syringe to evaporate the solvent and spread the film. This can be problematic if the 3-in-1 syringe is contaminated with water, which can be checked by blowing air from the syringe into a tissue. Common errors when

applying dentine-bonding agents include displacement of the agent with over enthusiastic use of the 3-in-1 syringe by the operator or assistant and incomplete evaporation of the solvent. It is recommended that the high-volume suction be directed so that a stream of air over the preparation evaporates the solvent.

If pulpal exposure or near exposure is suspected, then hard-setting calcium hydroxide cement should be used as described above as a direct or indirect pulp-capping agent. It is important to minimise the extent and thickness of the hard-setting calcium hydroxide cement, as extensive application of the material will limit the area of dentine available for bonding.

It has always been held that eugenol-containing restorative materials are contraindicated as liners for resin-composite restorations and temporary restorations for resin-bonded indirect restorations. This is because the eugenol is absorbed into the resin-composite restorative material or retained in the dentinal tubules, resulting in plasticising of the monomer and subsequent softening and discoloration of the resin-composite restoration and/or luting cement. The issue of residual eugenol in dentinal tubules has recently been investigated and it has been shown that the routine use of an etchant on dentine will remove residual eugenol from the dentinal tubules. Although the use of eugenol-containing liners is somewhat obsolete, it is now possible to use eugenol-containing temporary cements for temporisation of preparations destined to be restored with a resin-bonded restoration.

Recommended Reading

Hilton TJ. Cavity sealers, liners and bases: Current philosophies and indications for use. Oper Dent 1996;21:134-146.

Chapter 6

Minimising the Effects of Further Operative Intervention. Replace, Repair or Refurbish Failing Restorations?

Aim

Managing a failing restoration is a common clinical situation. The dilemma is often to decide which restorations require replacement and which would benefit from repair or refurbishment procedures. The aim of this section is to outline objective criteria to assist the practitioner in making these decisions. A further aim is for the practitioner to understand why restorations fail and so prevent future failures and improve outcomes.

Outcome

At the end of this section practitioners will be able to diagnose the reason that a restoration is failing and recognise restorations that can be repaired, refurbished or require replacement, and be familiar with the operative techniques associated with these procedures.

Introduction

Dental schools have, until recently, taught that restorations which did not meet certain specific criteria should be completely replaced along with any associated base and/or liner. This "drill-and-fill" philosophy, based on a mechanistic rather than a scientific approach to the operative management of dental caries, is flawed and can no longer be justified. The criteria used to assess the need to replace a restoration have not been based on evidence but upon the erroneous assumption that all marginal and interfacial defects, however small, are associated with the percolation of oral fluids along the tooth restoration interface, and that this leads inevitably to secondary caries. Consequently, practitioners in the UK spend about 50% of their chairside time replacing direct restorations that are deemed to have failed in clinical service. The reasons most commonly cited for replacing a direct restoration are as follows:
- secondary caries as diagnosed clinically
- marginal defects

- bulk fracture of the restoration
- fracture of adjacent tooth tissue
- marginal staining or restoration discolouration
- marginal excesses or overhangs
- wear.

Whilst some restorations will inevitably require replacement, it is suggested that many restorations – and not least the patient – would benefit from repair and/or refurbishment procedures. It is likely that many restorations in low-caries-risk individuals have needlessly been replaced when a less interventive approach could have been applied.

Each time restorations are replaced more tooth tissue is inevitably lost as preparations increase in size and progressively become more invasive. This has an adverse effect on the dental pulp and ultimately the restored unit if the restorative staircase is followed to its ultimate conclusion. It is clearly preferable, therefore, to repair, refurbish and maintain restorations wherever possible.

Until recently, repair and refurbishment of restorations has been thought of as substandard or less than optimal care. Anecdotally, there is evidence that practitioners repair and maintain restorations on a regular basis. There is, however, little information to assist practitioners in identifying restorations that would benefit from repair or refurbishment and very little about the operative procedures associated with these techniques, let alone information about the longevity of restorations repaired in this way.

Criteria for Repair and/or Refurbishment

The selection of restorations that would benefit from repair and/or refurbishment as opposed to complete restoration replacement is based on an assessment of patient-centred and tooth-specific criteria (Fig 6-1).

Patient-centred Criteria

Motivated and informed patients who attend on a regular basis, and in whom restorations can be monitored regularly, are good candidates for restoration repair and/or refurbishment procedures. Patients, who have complex medical histories or limited cooperation owing to learning difficulties, where treatment times and the nature of such interventions should be limited in terms of time and complexity, are especially suitable for repair and/or refur-

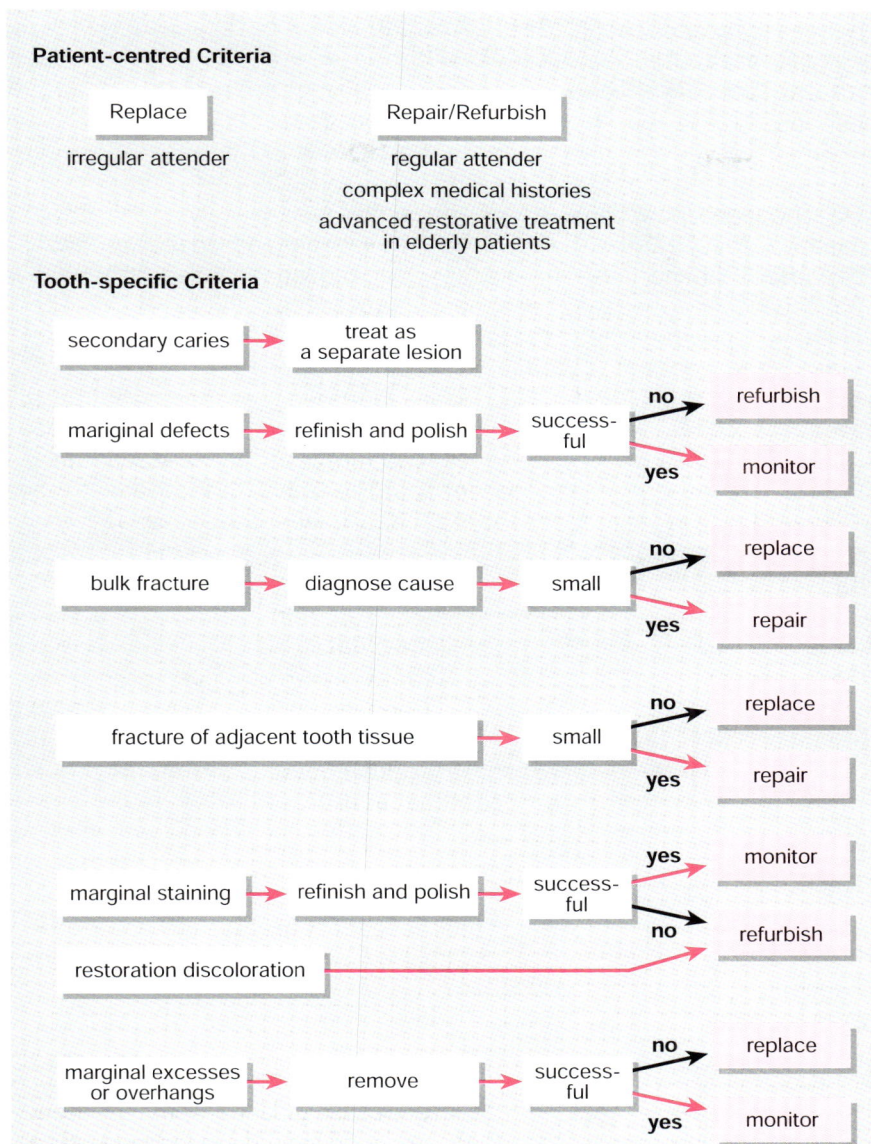

Fig 6-1 Algorithm for repairing, refurbishing and replacing restorations.

bishment procedures. Refurbishment procedures (for example, those applied to stained and/or discoloured resin-composite restorations in anterior teeth) can be accomplished in short treatment times frequently obviating the need for local anaesthesia. This can be particularly advantageous for all patients, but especially those with complex medical histories.

The management of failing advanced restorative dentistry in elderly patients is particularly problematic. Replacement of extensive reconstructions in these patients can lead to management difficulties, not least the possibility of not being able to remake the restorations or prejudicing the vitality of strategic abutment teeth. Repair, particularly of extensive reconstructions, should be encouraged in these patients wherever possible.

It is essential that patients understand the nature of repair and/or refurbishment procedures and how these procedures differ from restoration replacement procedures. In obtaining informed consent for repair and/or refurbishment procedures it is necessary to outline the disadvantages of replacement strategies in terms of their effect on the longevity of the restored unit. Similarly, the advantages of repair and refurbishment strategies in terms of the preservation of tooth tissue and their minimally interventive nature should be outlined. Further research into the prognosis and longevity of repaired and refurbished restorations is needed further to inform consent to repair and refurbishment procedures.

Patients who opt for repair and refurbishment procedures will in essence have a different pattern of care compared with those who opt for restoration replacement: regular visits for short, minimally interventive procedures, with occasional replacement procedures, as opposed to fewer, more infrequent visits, where interventions are limited to replacement procedures. It is sensible, therefore, to limit repair and refurbishment procedures to patients who attend on a regular basis.

Tooth-specific Criteria

It is important to accept that not all marginal defects in restorations require repair. Similarly, not all discoloured resin-composite restorations will require refurbishment. It is prudent to monitor such defects and not intervene until the patient is concerned, for example, about the aesthetics of an anterior tooth or where a marginal defect is causing food packing, sensitivity, soft tissue trauma, or caries is suspected.

The clinical presentations usually cited for replacing a restoration, along with how to prevent these failures and alternative management strategies, will be discussed in the next section.

Secondary caries

Caries (secondary) adjacent to the margin of a restoration should be treated as a primary lesion in its own right. As with all patients who present with a new lesion, preventive measures should be initiated primarily followed by operative intervention as and when the lesion is shown to be active and progressing into dentine and/or cavitation has occurred. Operative intervention should be limited to managing the lesion as minimally as possible, coupled with removal of the adjacent restoration only when its presence hinders successful management of the primary lesion in terms of access for effective caries removal. The need to remove all deep caries in modern-day operative dentistry has, however, been questioned, particularly when a restorative material is placed that adequately seals the preparation margins. It is suggested that the inability of amalgam to seal the margins of a preparation limits its use in this and other situations. New lesions suggest that the patient:

- is not complying with prescribed preventive regimes.
- has changed his/her consumption and frequency of consumption of fermentable carbohydrates (i.e. the diet is more cariogenic).

It is prudent to address these issues before proceeding to definitive treatment of caries.

Marginal defects

Visible marginal defects, which must not be confused with secondary caries, can often be removed with finishing and polishing procedures. Minimal defects on the occlusal surfaces of posterior teeth can be monitored and intervention reserved until there is clinical evidence of plaque accumulation and food stagnation. Marginal defects in anterior resin–composite restorations are more problematical because of their tendency to pick up exogenous stain. Finishing and polishing procedures, coupled with refurbishment of the restoration if required, are usually effective at removing this, and it is a good way to approach the restoration in the first instance, although it is not always successful (Figs 6-2–6-4). Marginal defects of direct restorations are likely to be due to one, or a combination, of the following factors:

- Inadequate or incorrect marginal preparation. For example, bevelling of occlusal preparations for resin composites or excessively acute or obtuse cavosurface margins for amalgam restorations with subsequent marginal fracture of the restorative material and/or unsupported enamel under occlusal loading.

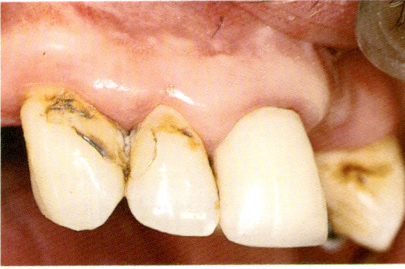

Fig 6-2 Stained resin composites with marginal defects in 13 and 12.

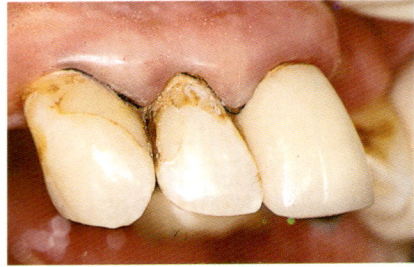

Fig 6-3 Persistent marginal defects after refinishing.

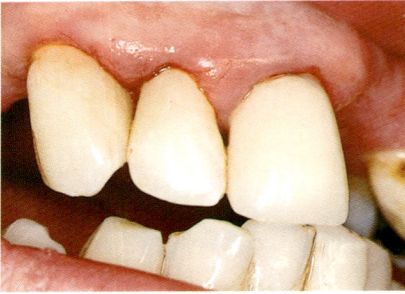

Fig 6-4 Replacement composites in 13 and 12.

- Fracture of overcontoured restorative material at the preparation margin particularly if the preparation margin is placed in an occlusal contact area.
- Poor adaptation of the restorative material during restoration placement.

Bulk fracture

When a patient presents with bulk fracture of a restoration, it is important to diagnose the reason for failure before considering treatment options. Bulk fracture of a restoration, particularly soon after restoration placement, is probably due to excess occlusal loading of a normally contoured restoration – possibly with preparation margins in occlusal contact areas or normal occlusal loading and over contouring of the restoration at placement. Bulk fracture of a restoration after years of clinical service is likely to be due to stress fatigue of the material. The treatment for a bulk fracture of a restoration is usually confined to the following:

- Direct restoration of the defect, most commonly with the same restorative material either using a dentine-bonding agent with resin-composite restorations or by keying the restoration into the remaining restorative

material, as in the repairing of amalgam restorations
- Larger bulk fractures may require restoration replacement and the prescription of a partial or full-coverage indirect restoration.

Prevention of bulk fracture of restorations is best achieved by:
- Assessing the patient's occlusion at restoration placement to include the use of articulating paper at the preparation and finishing stage.
- Not placing preparation margins in static or dynamic occlusal contact areas.
- Limiting the use of resin composite to small–medium occlusal and proximal preparations in premolar and permanent molar teeth.

Fracture of adjacent tooth tissue
Fracture of tooth tissue adjacent to a restoration is most likely due to:
- secondary caries undermining adjacent tooth tissue, with subsequent fracture
- unsupported tooth tissue fracturing under occlusal loading. This is common with amalgam restorations where the restoration does not support undermined tooth tissue at the margins of the preparation
- bulk curing of resin composite in large preparations with unsupported cusps. For example, large MOD preparations in premolar teeth, especially those previously restored with amalgam where undercuts have been previously placed with inverted cone burs
- loss of canine guidance
- bruxism or atypical occlusal loading
- recurrent trauma of anterior teeth.

Fracture of tooth tissue adjacent to a restoration is prevented by:
- use of preventive regimes alongside restorative therapy
- correct preparation design where unsupported tooth tissue is removed in preparations designed to be restored with amalgam
- use of adhesive materials that reinforce weakened tooth tissue (for example, resin composite or use of a bonded amalgam)
- use of an incremental placement technique coupled with a soft-start polymerisation technique for placing resin-composite restorations
- assessing the patient's occlusion at restoration placement to include the use of articulating paper at the preparation and finishing stages to ensure the restoration conforms to the patient's occlusal scheme
- not placing preparation margins in occlusal contact areas
- prescription of a mouth guard for patients who are involved in contact sports

- selective use of indirect restorations, specifically gold, resin composite or ceramic onlays to protect weakened cusps
- night guards in clenchers and bruxists.

Marginal staining or restoration discolouration

Staining of restoration margins is commonly seen in resin composite restorations and discolouration of the restoration itself exclusively with tooth-coloured restorative materials. Marginal staining is usually indicative of poor marginal adaptation of the restorative material, which can be due to the following:

- Inadequate etching of the marginal enamel of the preparation.
- Incorrect application of the dentine–bonding agent (for example, excessive drying with the three-in-one syringe, which displaces the bonding agent and/or thins it excessively).
- Poor adaptation of the restorative material at placement, with subsequent fracture of any marginal excesses in clinical service.
- Bulk curing of the material with polymerisation contraction stresses exceeding the tensile strength of the dentine–bonding agent, which results in interfacial gap formation.
- Smoking or excessive consumption of black tea or coffee.

Restorations with marginal staining are very suitable for refinishing procedures and, when the restoration itself is discoloured, refurbishment procedures.

Poor marginal adaptation and subsequent marginal staining can be prevented by:

- fine finishing of preparation margins
- use of etchant and dentine–bonding agents according to the manufacturer's directions for use
- gentle drying of dentine–bonding agents to evaporate the solvent, using a gentle stream of air from the three-in-one syringe, or preferably high-volume suction. It is sensible to agitate the dentine–bonding agent during this process if it is a sixth-generation dentin-bonding agent
- use of an appropriately contoured matrix band when proximal preparations are restored
- careful placement, finishing and polishing techniques. For resin composites the use of finishing tips that selectively remove resin composite rather than enamel are recommended
- use of an incremental placement technique coupled with a soft-start polymerisation technique for resin-composite restorations.

Marginal excesses or overhangs

Marginal excesses and/or overhangs of restorative materials acting as plaque-retention factors can be associated with localised periodontal defects, although this is less likely in patients with good plaque control. The presence of marginal excesses and overhangs inhibits good oral hygiene and encourages food stagnation. Marginal excesses and overhangs result from:

- Poor adaptation of the matrix band when proximal restorations are placed.
- Omitting to use a wedge, or inappropriate use of a wedge, in conjunction with a matrix band.
- Excessive force being used when placing and adapting the restorative material to the preparation.
- Failure to remove excess material before it has set in the case of amalgam restorations.
- Inadequate finishing procedures.

It is possible to remove marginal excesses or overhangs by selective use of:
- finishing and polishing strips
- ultrasonic scalers
- reciprocating handpieces with special tips (Figs 6-5–6-6)
- fine diamond finishing burs. However, there is a danger of damaging the adjacent tooth.

Restoration replacement will be required, however, if a combination of the above techniques is unsuccessful.

Marginal excesses and/or overhangs can be prevented by:
- use of a new matrix band for each procedure – ideally a disposable system coupled with the use of an interproximal wedge

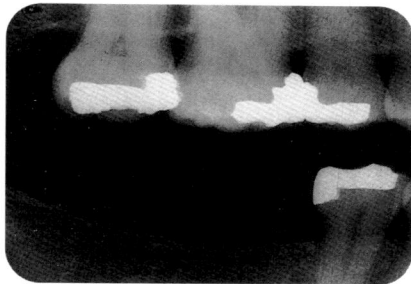

Fig 6-5 Radiograph of 16 featuring a mesial marginal excess of amalgam.

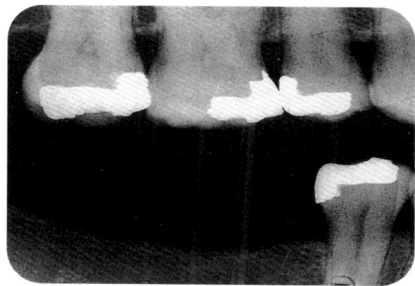

Fig 6-6 Radiograph of 16 after removal of marginal excess with a reciprocating handpiece.

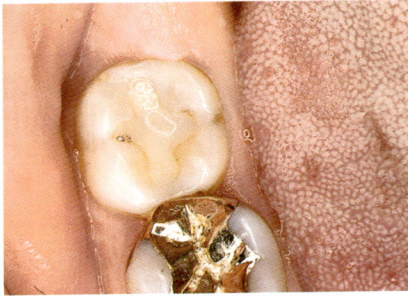

Fig 6-7 Resin composite in 48 showing occlusal wear after over 20 years of clinical service.

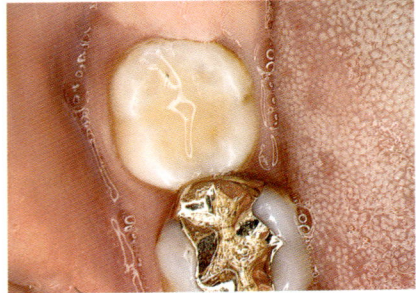

Fig 6-8 48 after veneering with resin composite.

- not using excessive packing forces when placing the restorative material. Resisting the temptation to pack and condense resin composite
- removal of excess material before the restorative material sets (for example, use of dental floss with amalgam restorations)
- judicious use of appropriate finishing procedures.

Wear
Much research has gone into the wear of resin composites, yet few require replacement solely because of excess wear. Veneering the worn surface of the restoration with resin composite would be a more appropriate procedure, although little is known about the reliability of bonding new increments of resin composite to clinically aged resin composite materials (Figs 6-7–6-8). Residual monomer in resin composites cured with a halogen lamp allows for bonding of new increments of resin composite material at a later date. Whether this will be the case with materials cured with curing strategies designed to increase monomer conversion rates remains to be seen.

Clinical Procedures

Repair
The clinical procedures for the repair of restorations are as follows (Fig 6-9–6-12):
- Local analgesia, if required.
- Isolation of the tooth with rubber dam.
- Access to caries, if present, established with a bur or, ideally, a safe-sided ultrasonic tip.
- Removal of the surface of the adjacent restorative material to provide a

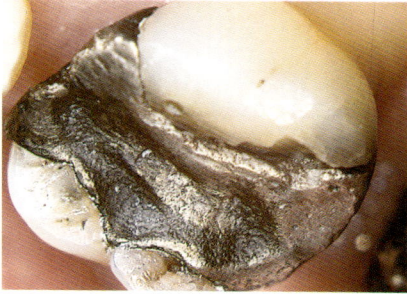

Fig 6-9 Amalgam in 16 featuring marginal deficiency.

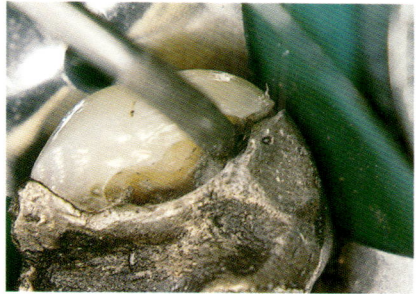

Fig 6-10 Preparation of 16 with sonic tips.

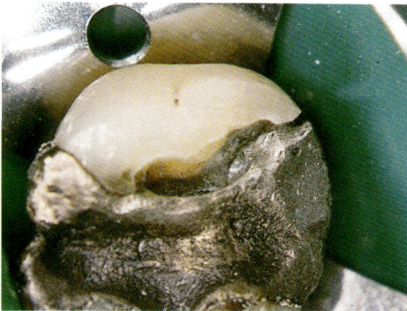

Fig 6-11 Completed preparation of 16.

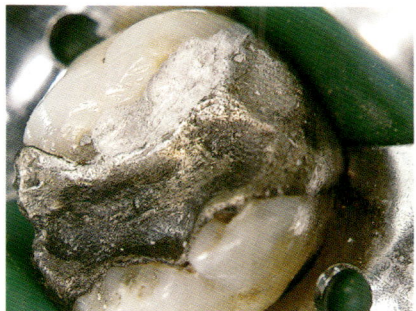

Fig 6-12 Amalgam repair placed in 16, which requires final finishing on review.

fresh surface to bond onto, or pack against in the case of amalgam. Surface treatment with an intra-oral sandblaster is useful to treat the surfaces of cast restorations needing marginal repair prior to bonding. Do not use a sandblaster on amalgam restorations, as it is likely to liberate aerosols of mercury.

- Inclusion of undercut or keys into adjacent restorative material to retain amalgam repairs. Please note it is a disadvantage of using amalgam for repair procedures that it is necessarily more destructive than using resin composite.
- Pulp protection, if required, according to contemporary regimes.
- Placement of the repair taking care to adapt it well to the preparation.
- Appropriate finishing and polishing procedures.
- Subsequent monitoring and review.

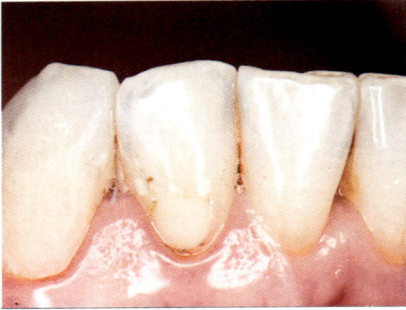

Fig 6-13 Stained resin composite restoration in 42.

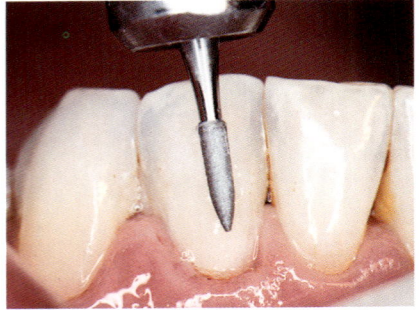

Fig 6-14 Stain removed with fine particle water-cooled diamond bur.

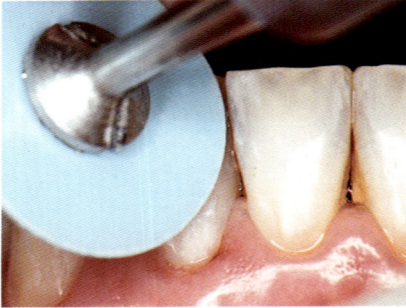

Fig 6-15 Polishing with a flexible disk.

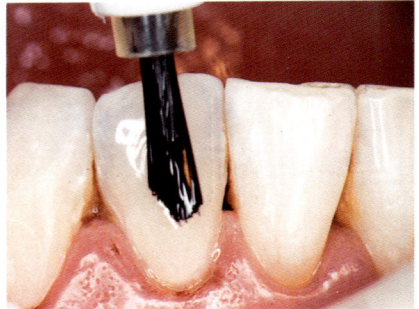

Fig 6-16 Application of unfilled resin to seal the restoration.

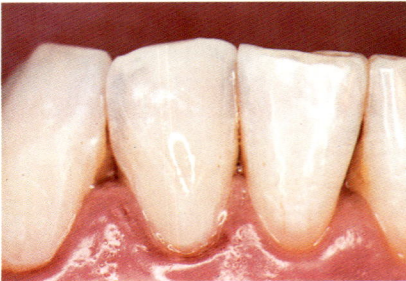

Fig 6-17 Completed refurbishment procedure.

Refurbishment

The clinical procedures for the refurbishment of a restoration, which will usually be for a resin-composite restoration, are as follows (Figs 6-13–6-17):

- If a posterior resin composite is to be refurbished because the surface of the restoration is worn, it is sensible to check the occlusion, as the opposing tooth may have over-erupted. If this has happened it may be necessary judiciously to reduce the opposing cusp before the restoration is refurbished.
- Local analgesia, if required.
- Isolation of the tooth with rubber dam.
- Cleaning the tooth with a slurry of pumice.
- Removal of the surface of the discoloured and/or stained restorative material to provide a fresh surface to bond onto. It is suggested around 1 mm of material is removed. Commonly, stained restorations will only require refinishing and polishing, with application of a bonding resin to reseal the restoration, and it might be sensible to start with refinishing and polishing with progression to a refurbishment procedure, if indicated.
- Bevelling of the occlusal margins is not appropriate, although a bevel on the margins of anterior proximal restorations is recommended.
- Etching of the enamel at the margins of the preparation.
- Application of a bonding agent, according to the directions for use.
- Incremental application of resin composite, with each increment individually cured for 40 seconds.
- Finishing and polishing procedures as required.
- Final application of bonding resin to seal the restoration surface.

Recommended Reading

Wilson NHF, Setcos JC, Brunton PA. Replacement or Repair of Dental Restorations. In: Wilson NHF, Roulet J-F, Fuzzi M (Eds.) Advances in Operative Dentistry. Vol 2: Challenges for the Future. Chicago: Quintessence, 2001.

Chapter 7

Notes on the Aetiology and Operative Management of Non-carious Tooth Tissue Loss. Erosion, Attrition or Abrasion?

Aim

As caries experience generally declines and improvements in the treatment and management of periodontal disease continue, the population are retaining more functional natural teeth. As a consequence, practitioners are seeing more patients with non-carious tooth tissue loss, the treatment for which can be complex in its advanced stages. The aim of this section is to alert practitioners to the early signs of non-carious tooth tissue loss and to consider preventive regimes and early operative management of the condition with direct restorative materials.

Outcome

On completion of this section practitioners will be able to diagnose non-carious tooth tissue loss (NCTTL) in its early stages and be familiar with the use of direct restorative materials in the early management of NCTTL.

Introduction

NCTTL is defined as tooth tissue or surface loss due to a disease process other than dental caries. It is often termed tooth wear, which is technically a misleading term as it implies a purely abrasive basis for the disease. NCTTL is due to erosion, abrasion or attrition. *Abrasion* is defined as: "an abnormal wearing away of a substance or structure by a mechanical process". *Attrition* is defined as: "loss of tooth substance or of a restoration as a result of mastication or of occlusal or proximal contact between the teeth". *Erosion* is defined as: "progressive loss of hard dental tissues by an acidic chemical process without bacterial action".

These pathological processes rarely occur in isolation. NCTTL is therefore considered to be multifactorial in nature. As the lost tissues are not replaced, the effects of the disease process are therefore cumulative and irreversible.

The UK has an increasingly ageing dentate population, with an average life expectancy of eighty (plus) years. The prevalence of NCTTL has increased considerably in recent years and underlying trends indicate that it will continue to do so; consequently, the cumulative effects of NCTTL will therefore present a considerable restorative management problem in the future.

Abrasion

This is essentially mechanical wear of tooth surfaces by extraneous agents and four types have been identified. *Cervical abrasion,* also termed "abfraction", is characterised by a v-shaped groove at the cervical margin of anterior and posterior teeth (Fig 7-1). It is usually more prominent on canines and premolars. There are many views as to the aetiology of this type of lesion, which include:

- Stress corrosion. This occurs when erosive agents contact teeth, which vertically barrel under occlusal loading.
- Horizontal toothbrushing. The absence of a smear layer, the presence of abrasion in individuals who don't brush their teeth, and the presence of lesions subgingivally make this theory untenable.

The above theories have largely been superseded by the concept of "abfraction". This theory suggests that flexure of a tooth during occlusal loading causes micro-fractures in the cervical enamel with subsequent cavitation. Although this is held to be the cause it has never been demonstrated in a scientific study. It also does not explain why teeth which are not in occlusion still develop lesions

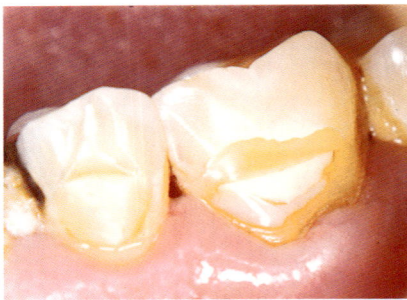

Fig 7-1 36 featuring an abfraction lesion.

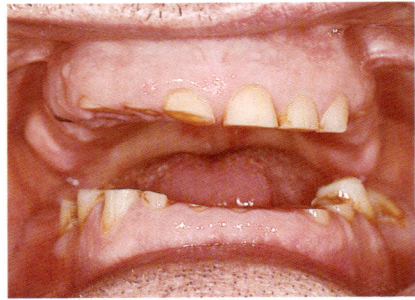

Fig 7-2 Attrition.

Habitual abrasion has a variable clinical presentation, which is dependent on the causative factor. Classic and often-quoted examples include: pipe smoking and hairgrips. *Iatrogenic abrasion* includes the grinding of opposing teeth to accommodate restorations. Note that unglazed ceramic crowns also cause abrasion of the opposing teeth. Although the newer ceramic systems have similar wear rates to that of enamel, metal occlusal surfaces for posterior indirect porcelain fused to metal restorations are still to be preferred. Historically, *industrial abrasion* has also been described but is less common owing to better control of industrial environments. It was principally seen in industrial settings where abrasive particles were present in the atmosphere.

Attrition

The clinical features include (Fig 7-2):

- shortening of crowns with flattening of occlusal surfaces and incisal edges
- exposure of dentine and secondary dentine
- worn surfaces of opposing teeth that fit together accurately
- overgrowth of alveolar processes, more correctly termed dento-alveolar compensation.

The aetiology of attrition is complex and poorly understood. A parafunctional habit as a result of a difference between the retruded contact position and intercuspal position is probably the commonest cause. Tradition presupposes that the lack of posterior teeth (support) may be responsible for attrition of the anterior teeth. There is no evidence to support this theory and the proprioceptive fibres of the anterior teeth should prevent excessive loading. The nature of the process is so slow that secondary dentine forms and thus sensitivity is not usually part of the clinical picture. Sensitivity precludes attrition as an aetiological factor. However, attrition superimposed on erosion or vice versa could well present with sensitivity.

Two types of attrition have been described. *Physiological attrition* is defined as gradual and regular loss of tooth substance as a result of "normal" mastication. Attrition confined to local areas or specific groups of teeth, caused by abnormal function, is termed *pathological attrition*.

Erosion

The clinical features of erosion depend upon the source of the erosive agent. *Extrinsic* erosion due to acid present in the diet will on the whole affect the labial surface of the anterior teeth and to a lesser extent the occlusal surfaces of the lower permanent molars (Fig 7-3). *Intrinsic* erosion due to acid regur-

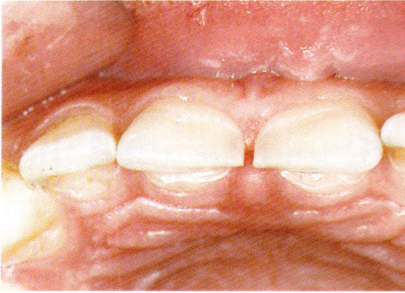

Fig 7-3 Extrinsic erosion.

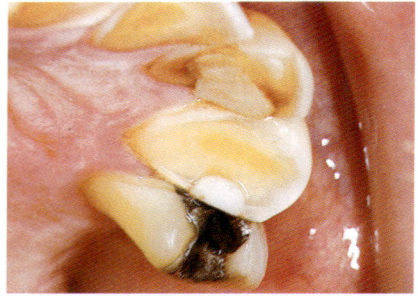

Fig 7-4 Intrinsic erosion.

gitation (gastric acid) will usually affect the palatal surfaces of the upper teeth and on occasion the occlusal surfaces of the lower permanent molars (Fig 7-4). It would be helpful if the aetiological basis for erosion was so clear cut. Anorexic patients are often dehydrated due to starvation, use of laxatives and diuretics. As a consequence, they consume carbonated drinks and fruit juice to quench their thirst, which in turn produce labial erosion. This can confuse matters further when attempting to identify an aetiological cause. Anxiolytics prescribed for the treatment of anorexia nervosa can produce xerostomia (dry mouth) and can potentiate the erosive process due to reduced salivary buffering. It must be emphasised again that attrition and abrasion can exacerbate the effects of erosion.

Erosion is therefore classified according to the source of the erosive acid (see Fig 7-5). The clinical features of erosion include:

- Loss of surface characteristics, giving a smooth enamel surface (very unlike etched enamel, which has a rough appearance). Very often the cervical area of the tooth is most severely affected. This has lead to the suggestion that erosion is implicated in the formation of cervical cavities.
- Labial furrows with the enamel surface having a criss-crossed appearance.
- Palatal hollows usually bearing no relationship to the occlusal relationship. This would exclude attrition as the cause.
- Reduction in the height of the clinical crown in severe cases.
- Cupping of lower molar cusp tips.
- Palatal chipping of upper incisal edges.
- "Proud" restorations.

Patients with extrinsic erosion, which is dietary in nature, will commonly have a history of excessive consumption of the following:

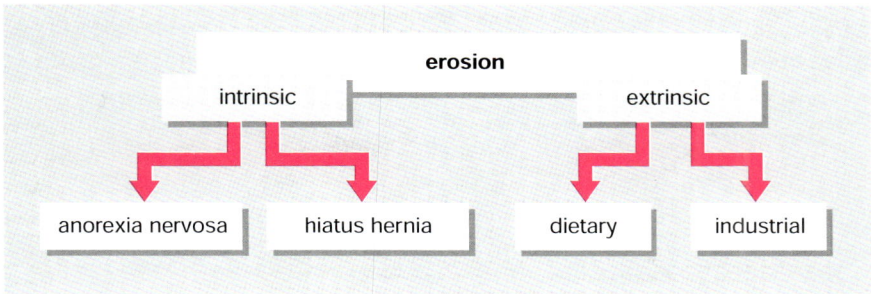

Fig 7-5 Classification of erosion according to the source of the erosive acid.

- citrus and fruit juices
- carbonated drinks (pH 2–3)
- alcohol, specifically white wine
- citrus-based fruit teas.

Exposure to extrinsic acid may well occur as a result of frequent swimming in heavily chlorinated water. This is likely to affect swimming instructors and professional athletes, particularly if associated with excessive consumption of "sports drinks".

Historically, *industrial erosion* has been described in workers in battery and electrolytic zinc factories: acidic particles in the atmosphere were responsible for the erosion. Industrial erosion is unlikely to be seen in the UK today because of very explicit health and safety legislation.

Intrinsic erosion is due to gastric acid reflux or vomiting, which can occur in the following conditions:

Reflux
- symptomatic or asymptomatic gastro–oesophageal reflux
- gastric ulceration
- hiatus hernia
- alcohol abuse.

Vomiting
- anorexia nervosa
- bulimia nervosa (Note: these patients are usually within ± 15% of their normal weight)
- pregnancy.

A condition known as perimylolysis has been described. This condition produces loss of lingual enamel and dentine due to acid regurgitation aggravated by circular movements of the tongue. Stress reflux syndrome has also been described. It usually affects young affluent members of the enterprise culture with reflux occurring during the day and often at work. The regurgitated stomach contents are held in the mouth before being swallowed again. This syndrome produces an atypical pattern of erosion with the buccal surfaces of the lower posterior teeth affected. It has been suggested that axial loading of the teeth may be a factor as well.

Clinical Consequences

The clinical consequences of NCTTL include:
- poor aesthetics
- impaired function
- lack of occlusal stability
- pain, discomfort and sensitivity.

Monitoring is an integral part of the treatment of NCTTL. A suitable method of quantifying the degree of NCTTL experienced by a patient, and that can be repeated subsequently, is therefore required. Many methods of classification, too numerous to cover comprehensively, have been described in the literature. The most often used is that described by Smith and Knight (1984). This index is very useful for research. However, a more pragmatic index is urgently required for practitioners. Until such time, serial study casts are very helpful in monitoring tooth wear.

Management of NCTTL

The management of NCTTL involves four stages:
  I. Identify the cause and assess the long-term prognosis for the patient's dentition.
  II. Institute preventive measures and try to control the problem.
  III. Monitor the disease process.
  IV. Operative treatment if required.

Prevention of Further NCTTL

It is very important that the correct aetiological factor is identified if appropriate preventive measures are to be implemented. You may have to liaise with the patient's medical practitioner, particularly if you suspect intrinsic

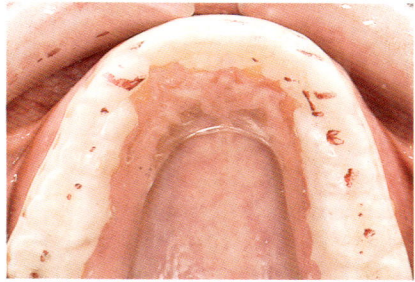

Fig 7-6 Stabilization splint.

erosion as being the cause of the NCTTL. It is helpful to explain to your medical colleague, in the referral letter, the association between eating disorders, reflux, etc. and NCTTL. It is also important to emphasise that reflux can often be asymptomatic and NCTTL can be the first sign of an underlying problem. A dietary history will be required if you suspect an extrinsic erosive cause and counselling the patient with regard to their dietary habits may be necessary.

An acrylic splint, in the form of a stabilisation splint, may be necessary to protect the dentition from further damage due to attrition and this is frequently the only treatment required. Patient compliance with splint wear can be problematical. It may also be used as a diagnostic aid, particularly if an increase in the occlusal vertical dimension is planned subsequently. If abnormal occlusal loading is identified as an aetiological factor this will also need to be corrected, but only after a period of splint wear.

The most helpful splint in the management and diagnosis of patients with tooth wear is a hard acrylic splint in the form of a stabilisation splint. This splint is designed to have the following features (Fig 7-6):
• even contact of all teeth in centric relation (RCP).
• protrusive and excursive guidance.
• no non-working interferences.

To produce a stabilisation splint for a patient the laboratory will need the following:
• full arch impressions
• facebow record
• centric and relation record.

The splint will need to be relined with cold-cure acrylic resin to improve the retention of the appliance, and occlusal adjustment will typically be required. Frequently, this is the only treatment required to prevent further tooth tissue loss.

If you have a patient who has a history of recurrent vomiting (for example, as in anorexia nervosa), advise the patient not to brush their teeth after vomiting. This is because tooth brushing will further abrade the eroded tooth tissue. Instead, counsel your patient to rinse with one of the following:
- 0.05% sodium fluoride rinse
- alkaline mineral water.

These will neutralise the effects of the acid, prevent further erosion and decrease subsequent sensitivity.

Monitoring of NCTTL

If NCTTL is recognised in its early stages and appropriate preventive advice is given, frequently no further treatment will be required. It is helpful to monitor these cases for evidence of further signs of disease activity. The best way to do this is to take baseline study casts and photographs and repeat this at intervals to see if the NCTTL is progressing. Other indicators of continuing NCTTL include ongoing sensitivity, along with metallic restorations becoming proud of the adjacent tooth tissue in patients where erosion is suspected to be the primary cause of the NCTTL.

Treatment of NCTTL

The management of patients with severe NCTTL can be very complex and destructive. Simple operative treatment, which can be very effective, can include the following:
- desensitisation treatments
- simple restorations
- canine risers.

Desensitisation treatments
The new dentine-bonding agents have changed the treatment of dentine hypersensitivity considerably. Until relatively recently, the only treatment available to practitioners comprised fluoride gels and/or desensitising toothpastes. Neither of these treatments gave predictable results in the long term. The use of fifth- and sixth-generation dentine-bonding agents, especially those incorporating filler particles, offers practitioners a predictable treatment for dentine hypersensitivity (Fig 7-7). The treatment is applied with-

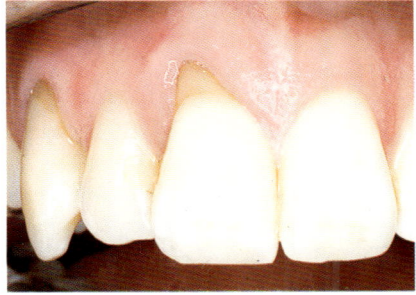

Fig 7-7 11 and 13 featuring buccal dentine hypersensitivity.

out local anaesthesia, is painless and typically requires additional applications every six months. The use of dentine-bonding agents in this way in minimal non-carious cervical lesions frequently obviates the need for a restoration. Restoration of non-carious cervical lesions should only be undertaken if the lesion is active, unaesthetic or troublesome to the patient. Restorations have a finite lifespan and they will require replacement at periodic intervals, possibly trapping the patient into a placement–replacement cycle for the rest of their lives.

A dentine-bonding agent that contains the antimicrobial triclosan is now available for the treatment of sensitive, exposed cervical dentine. The antimicrobial is incorporated to prevent root caries.

Simple restorations
Resin-bonded tooth-coloured restorations are increasingly used to restore NCTTL. It is now recognized that resin composite is useful for restoring defects caused by erosion and attrition. The use of resin composite in this way is helpful for diagnostic purposes (for example, to test a patient's tolerance to an increase in the vertical dimension of occlusion). Direct composite restorations can be used to restore canine guidance in the form of canine risers and can also to have a "Dahl" type effect if the six anterior teeth are restored to treat palatal erosion at an increased vertical dimension of occlusion. The restorations can often be left as definite restorations with no further operative intervention being required.

Canine risers
Canine risers aim to re-establish canine guidance and posterior disclusion during mandibular excursion. They alter eccentric tooth contacts by changing the guidance angle on the canine without affecting the maximal intercuspal position or centric occlusion. They are increasingly made from direct

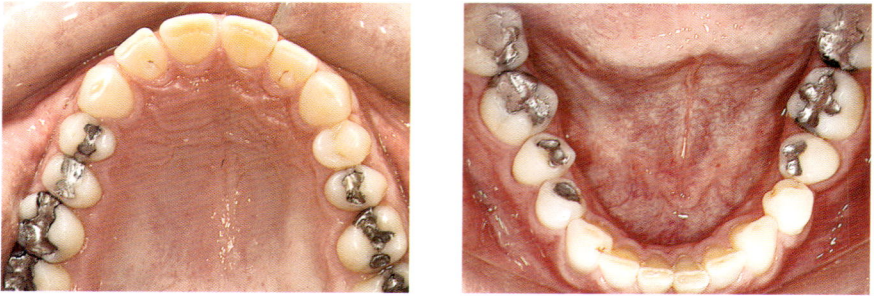

Fig 7-8 Patient showing occlusal wear due to bruxism and parafunction.

composite especially for diagnostic purposes. They have the advantage that their provision does not involve the extensive tooth preparation required to recreate anterior guidance with crowns. In addition, canine risers avoid the need for the patient to wear a removable appliance to control tooth wear associated with bruxism, or to provide lost anterior guidance.

The technique described is recommended for the treatment of cases of moderate tooth wear featuring an element of bruxism or parafunction and which have been treated successfully with a stabilization splint (Figs 7-6 and 7-8). For the technique to be successful, the canine teeth should be relatively sound, and have sufficient enamel in terms of quality and quantity to facilitate the bonding of resin composite in the form of a canine riser to the palatal surface. The canine teeth must be placed in the arch such that restoration of the palatal surface of the canine will establish a canine-guided occlusion. It is recommended that a resin composite canine riser be placed in the first instance both to confirm the patient's suitably for this form of treatment and further to aid diagnosis. Subject to satisfactory progress, the resin composite restoration can be converted to either metal or ceramic in due course, if required.

To place direct resin composite canine risers, local anaesthesia is not required. Resin composite is added to the palatal surface of the canines until even contact in centric relation at an increased vertical dimension of occlusion of approximately 1 mm is obtained. The risers should be designed to incorporate excursive contacts, which give immediate disclusion of the posterior teeth during excursive movements of the mandible (Fig 7-9).
The patient should be reviewed one week after placement and the occlusion monitored closely at monthly intervals until even posterior contact is

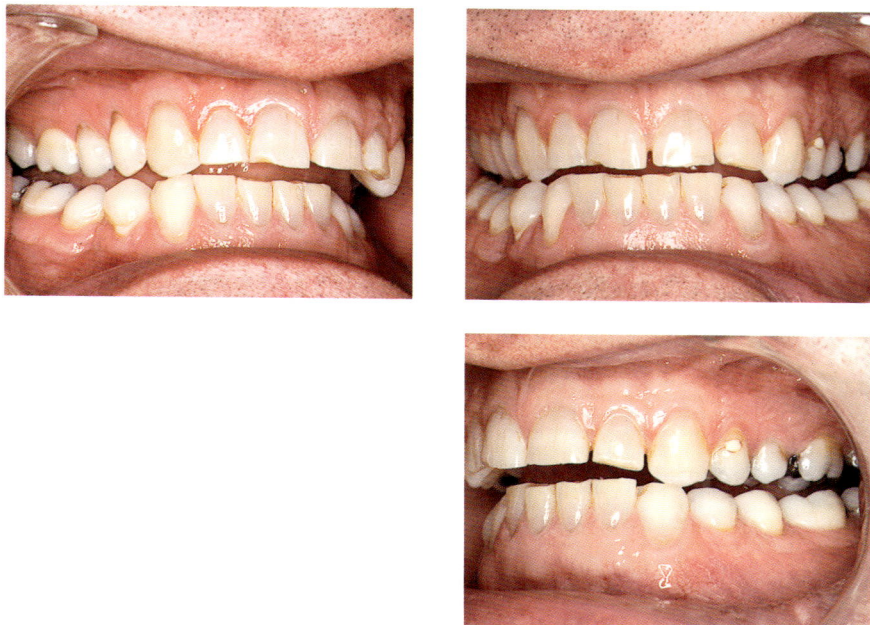

Fig 7-9 Patient after direct placement of resin composite canine risers.

established. The degree of wear of the resin composite must be monitored visually and/or with serial study casts. When there is evidence of excessive wear of the resin-composite canine riser, consideration should be given to placing a further restoration made from either ceramic or metal. If a metal riser will result with an unaesthetic show of metal at the tip of the canine, porcelain-fused-to-metal crowns can be placed on the upper canines. Care must be taken that the centric contacts and the first 2 mm of excursive guidance are planned to be on the metal surface.

Recommended Reading

Murray MC, Brunton PA, Osborne-Smith K, Wilson NHF. Canine risers: indications and techniques for their use. Eur J Prosthodont Rest Dent 2001;9:137-140.

Index

Quintessentials for General Dental Practitioners Series

in 36 volumes

Editor-in-Chief: Professor Nairn H F Wilson

The Quintessentials for General Dental Practitioners Series covers basic principles and key issues in all aspects of modern dental medicine. Each book can be read as a stand-alone volume or in conjunction with other books in the series.

Publication date, approximately

Oral Surgery and Oral Medicine, Editor: John G Meechan

Practical Dental Local Anaesthesia	available
Practical Oral Medicine	Spring 2004
Practical Conscious Sedation	Autumn 2003
Practical Surgical Dentistry	Spring 2004

Imaging, Editor: Keith Horner

Interpreting Dental Radiographs	available
Panoramic Radiology	Autumn 2003
Twenty-first Century Dental Imaging	Autumn 2004

Periodontology, Editor: Iain L C Chapple

Understanding Periodontal Diseases: Assessment and Diagnostic Procedures in Practice	available
Decision-Making for the Periodontal Team	Autumn 2003
Successful Periodontal Therapy – A Non-Surgical Approach	Autumn 2003
Periodontal Management of Children and Adolescents	Autumn 2003
Periodontal Medicine in Practice	Spring 2004

Implantology, Editor: Lloyd J Searson

Implants for the General Practitioner	available
Managing Orofacial Pain in General Dental Practice	Spring 2003

Endodontics, Editor: John M Whitworth

Rational Root Canal Treatment in Practice	available
Managing Endodontic Failure in Practice	Autumn 2003
Managing Dental Trauma in Practice	Autumn 2003
Managing the Vital Pulp in Practice	Autumn 2004

Prosthodontics, Editor: P Finbarr Allen

Teeth for Life for Older Adults	available
Complete Dentures – from Planning to Problem Solving	Autumn 2003
Removable Partial Dentures – A Systematic Approach	Autumn 2003
Fixed Prosthodontics for the General Dental Practitioner	Autumn 2003
Occlusion: A Theoretical and Team Approach	Autumn 2004

Operative Dentistry, Editor: Paul A Brunton

Decision-Making in Operative Dentistry	available
Applied Dental Materials in Operative Dentistry	Spring 2003
Aesthetic Dentistry	Autumn 2003
Successful Indirect Restorations in General Practice	Spring 2004

Paediatric Dentistry/Orthodontics, Editor: Marie Therese Hosey

Child Taming: How to Cope with Children in Dental Practice	Spring 2003
Paediatric Cariology	Autumn 2003
Treatment Planning for the Developing Dentition	Autumn 2003

General Dentistry and Practice Management, Editor: Raj Rattan

The Business of Dentistry	available
Risk Management in General Dental Practice	Spring 2003
Practice Management for the Dental Team	Autumn 2003
Application of Information Technology in General Dental Practice	Spring 2004
Quality Assurance in General Dental Practice	Autumn 2004
Evidence-Based Care in General Dental Practice	Spring 2005

Quintessence Publishing Co. Ltd., London